PRAISE FOR

Mating in C

"*Mating in Captivity* takes a hard line against one of the most time-honored institutions in human history: the sexless marriage. . . . It reads like a cross between the works of Jacques Lacan and *French Women Don't Get Fat*."
—*The New Yorker*

"As revelatory as it is straightforward . . . nicely accessible. . . . [Perel] offers the estranged modern couple a unique richness of experience."
—*Publishers Weekly*

"Perel tells us why intimacy can feel imprisoning and how we can embrace the erotic—without leaving home. Her writing is fresh and provocative, in a class by itself."
—Janis Abrahms Spring, Ph.D., author of
After the Affair: Healing the Pain and Rebuilding
Trust When a Partner Has Been Unfaithful

"Esther Perel is a fearless writer and thinker who will challenge your views about sex in a radical and fundamental way. She has the most original, edgy, intelligent, and high-spirited voice out there on passionless sex versus erotic vitality. She writes like a dream, making it nearly impossible to put down this book even when you want to."
—Harriet Lerner, Ph.D., author of *The Dance of Anger*

"Perel has written the first really engaging and provocative 'sex' book in years! With psychological sophistication and evocative prose, she reminds us what many of us would rather forget: to un-domesticate sex requires paying attention to our erotic imagination and moving beyond the security of the familiar but comfortable. An erotic sexual life is for those who want more than 'workable' sex. Perel tells us how to find it."
—Sandra Leiblum, Ph.D., Director,
Center for Sexual and Relationship Health,
Robert Wood Johnson Medical School

"Finally! A book that truly addresses the mystery of sustaining erotic desire in long term relationships. Esther Perel's *Mating in Captivity* is a brilliantly written, illuminating book about the conundrum that most couples face in relationship: how to keep the romantic spark glowing over a lifetime. Perel doesn't offer yet another sex manual; rather she engages us to be open to the magic and mystery of erotic exploration that's possible for couples. She shows the rich variety of ways couples can rekindle their romance when they rediscover their separateness, differences, and vulnerable yearnings with tenderness and curiosity. This is a book I would recommend to a couple for their honeymoon and a couple celebrating their fiftieth anniversary. It's a book I've asked my wife to read. And my sons. It's by my bedside. Consider having it by yours."
—David Treadway, Ph.D., author of
Intimacy, Change, and Other Therapeutic Mysteries

"Her advice is refreshingly counterintuitive." —Salon.com

"*Mating in Captivity* . . . articulates a poignant and unacknowledged modern crisis for the first time." —*Evening Standard* (UK)

"Perel says the kind of things that are so contrary to popular wisdom, they actually sound blasphemous—and yet, at precisely the same moment that you're being shocked by her, you're also acknowledging the validity of her ideas. Perel's ideas are . . . instantly familiar because they resonate deeply. It's all rather terrifying in its intuitiveness and its pure rightness." —*Observer* (UK)

"Perel's main point is that a happy marriage is a sexy one. . . . Far from being smug, Perel's position on the matter is almost survivalist."
—*Guardian* (UK)

"An elegant sociological study, complete with erudite literary and anthropological references." —*Daily Telegraph* (UK)

"Challenging the conventional wisdom, Esther Perel examines sexuality and eroticism as both independent of and yet intersecting with intimacy and commitment. *Mating in Captivity* is a significant contribution, as useful to clinicians as it is informative to the general public. Her clinical illustrations depict sophisticated clinical work in a manner that is lively and engaging." —Lewis Aron, Ph.D., Director,
New York University Postdoctoral Program
in Psychotherapy and Psychoanalysis

"An academic perspective on the deterioration of sex in relationships. . . . Perel offers insightful, progressive theories on how to put the play back into partnerships." —*Daily Record & Sunday Mail* (UK)

"Part sociological study, part voyeurism, and elegantly, if not erotically, written. . . . There's a tableau of sexual conundrums laid out in *Mating in Captivity* that covers most bases. You'll be sure to find yourself in there somewhere." —*Australian*

"A charming blend of wit and wisdom . . . this book will give you a fresh perspective on long-term love." —*Gold Coast Bulletin* (Australia)

"*Mating in Captivity* is a provocative look into the waning of sexual desire that often plagues couples in long-term relationships. This book serves as an excellent resource for the neophyte in the field of sex and couples therapy, serving to debunk some of the stereotypes that abound around sexual desire. Just as fitting for the professional, the book is an important source of information for the lay consumer wishing to add passion to his/her relationship." —Lori Brotto,
Journal of Sex and Marital Therapy

"[*Mating in Captivity*] makes fewer promises and raises thornier questions than any other how-to-improve-your-relationship book you've ever read, which is exactly why you should read this one. . . . [Perel] writes with worldliness and nuance and seems as comfortable drawing on Proust as from *Passionate Marriage*." —*Elle*

"Marriage feeling a little . . . passionless? In her new book [*Mating in Captivity*] New York therapist Esther Perel offers couples a battle plan for fighting sexual burnout." —*People*

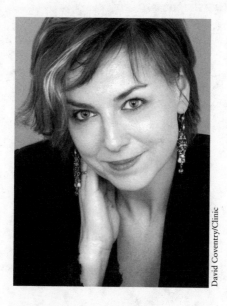

David Coventry/Clinic

About the Author

ESTHER PEREL is a psychotherapist with a private practice in New York City. She is on the faculty of the International Trauma Studies Program, affiliated with Columbia University; is a member of the American Family Therapy Academy; and has appeared on many television programs, including *The Oprah Winfrey Show*, *Good Day New York*, *CBS This Morning*, and *Women Aloud*. She lives in New York City with her husband and two children.

Mating in Captivity

Unlocking Erotic Intelligence

Esther Perel

HARPER

NEW YORK • LONDON • TORONTO • SYDNEY

HARPER

"Wild Things in Captivity," from *The Complete Poems of D. H. Lawrence* by D. H. Lawrence, edited by V. de Sola Pinto & F. W. Roberts, copyright © 1964, 1971 by Angelo Ravagli and C. M. Weekley, Executors of the Estate of Frieda Lawrence Ravagli. Used by permission of Viking Penguin, a division of Penguin Group (USA) Inc.

All names and identifying details of the individuals in this book have been changed to protect their privacy.

A hardcover edition of this book was published in 2006 by HarperCollins Publishers.

HarperCollins books may be purchased for educational, business, or sales promotional use. For information, please e-mail the Special Markets Department at SPsales@harpercollins.com.

FIRST HARPER PAPERBACK PUBLISHED 2007.

Designed by Nancy Singer Olaguera

The Library of Congress has catalogued the hardcover edition as follows:
    Perel, Esther
      Mating in captivity : reconciling the erotic and the domestic / Esther Perel.—1st ed.
        p.   cm.
      Includes bibliographical references and index.
      ISBN-10: 0-06-075363-3
      ISBN-13: 978-0-06-075363-4
        1. Sex and marriage. 2. Couples—Sexual behavior—Psychological aspects. 3. Sexual excitement. 4. Sexual desire disorders. 5. Man-woman relationships—Psychological aspects. I. Title.
      HQ734.P397 2006
      306.87—dc22   2006043533

ISBN: 978-0-06-075364-1 (pbk.)
ISBN-10: 0-06-075364-1 (pbk.)

24 25 26 27 28 LBC 54 53 52 51 50

To my parents, Sala Ferlegier and Icek Perel.
Their vitality lives on in me.

Acknowledgments

I NEVER WROTE A BOOK before. I thought I couldn't stand the solitude. To my surprise, I found I could bring my love of collaboration and midnight chats to the writing table. I tend to think in conversation—it's in speaking that my ideas emerge and take on clarity. Some people helped me talk, and others, write. I owe them so much, far beyond this modest tribute. Since we have been musing about love and sex for two years, let me simply say that every word sends a kiss of gratitude.

Sarah Manges, editor extraordinaire, you have been my compass. You have kept me on course when squalls of ideas threatened to knock me way off. Laura Blum, you levitated my prose. Not being a native English-speaker, I miss certain nuances of the language that your poetic flair always captures. Michele Scheinkman, I never know that an idea makes sense until you give it your seal of approval. Gail Winston, my editor at HarperCollins, you believed in me like a mother. You made me pick up my strewn thoughts and kept me jargon-free. Mary Wylie, when you edited the original article from which this book is drawn, "In Search of Erotic Intelligence: Reconciling Sensuality and Domesticity," did you know how far we would go? You often understood what I wanted to say before I did. Miriam Horn, you were the first person who gave some shape to the original article. Rich Simon, you set this whole thing in motion. A simple question in the spring of 2002, "What have you been thinking about lately?" prompted me to send you some loose ideas which, eleven versions later, ended in the pages of an on-the-cusp magazine, *The Psychotherapy Networker*. Things could have ended there, with an interesting article. But Tracy Brown, you were rummaging through the newsstands as only an enterprising agent knows how to do. You spotted the cover of the *Utne Reader*, which had reproduced my article from the *Networker* article. We instantly bonded, and began this amazing journey. I'm recommending you right and left. Ilana Berger, you introduced me to the world of sex therapy. You've been a mentor and a friend. Peter Fraenkel, since before day one you believed in this project. Michael Shernoff, by offering a gay perspective, you kept me from falling into heterosexual clichés. Patti Cohen and David Bornstein, I'm honored that you've welcomed me into your circle of writers. Deborah Gieringer, Sandy Petrey, and Katherine Frank, thank you for being such discerning readers and thinkers. Phillis Levin, you are my poetic muse. Shelly Kellner, you bring a wealth of organization to my chaos. Your research support was impeccable. Anya Strzemien, you spent hours listening to me on tape and then transcribing. Can we work together again? Miriam Baker, thank you for the wonderful metaphor of captivity.

There's no way to overstate the contribution of my patients. I'm honored by your trust in me. Thank you for letting me into your souls, and for allowing me to take your stories to enrich the life of others. Friends, too, please join the list. I can't name everyone who sat at my dinner table parsing out the complexities of desire, but you know who you are, and I can't thank you enough.

Jack Saul, we have been together nearly a quarter of a century. I know you appreciate my choice of topic! I wouldn't have been able to complete this project without your enduring support and enthusiasm. You stepped in whenever I stepped out. Adam, my older son, you are my computer whiz. It's meant so much to me that you've taken such an interest in my work even when my work has taken me elsewhere. Noam, my younger son, I promise you that when you come of age I'll be delighted to have you read my book.

WILD THINGS IN CAPTIVITY

Wild things in captivity
while they keep their own wild purity
won't breed, they mope, they die.

All men are in captivity,
active with captive activity,
and the best won't breed, though they don't know why.

The great cage of our domesticity
kills sex in a man, the simplicity
of desire is distorted and twisted awry.

And so, with bitter perversity,
gritting against the great adversity,
the young ones copulate, hate it, and want to cry.

Sex is a state of grace.
In a cage it can't take place.
Break the cage then, start in and try.

D. H. Lawrence

Contents

Introduction

THE STORY OF SEX IN committed modern couples often tells of a dwindling desire and includes a long list of sexual alibis, which claim to explain the inescapable death of eros. Recently, it seems, everyone from the morning news to the *New York Times* has weighed in on the topic. They warn us that too many couples are having infrequent sex even when the partners profess to love each other. Today's twosomes are too busy, too stressed, too involved in child rearing, and too tired for sex. And if all this isn't enough to dull their senses, then it's the antidepressants meant to alleviate the stress that set off the final unraveling. This is indeed an ironic development for the baby boomers who some thirty years ago ushered in a new age of sexual liberation. Now that these men and women and the generations who have followed can have as much sex as they want, they seem to have lost their desire for it.

Though I have no quarrel with the accuracy of these reports in the media—our lives are surely more stressful than they should be—it seems to me that in focusing almost exclusively on the frequency and quantity of sexual relations, they address only the most superficial reasons for the malaise so many couples are feeling. I think there's more to the story.

Psychologists, sex therapists, and social observers have long grappled with the Gordian knot of how to reconcile sexuality and domesticity. We're offered prolific advice on how to shop in the spice market to add additional flavors to committed sex. Languishing desire, we're coached, is a scheduling problem that can be fixed with better prioritizing and organizational skills; or it is a communication problem that can be ameliorated by verbally expressing precisely what we want sexually.

I'm less inclined toward a statistical approach to sex—whether you're still having it, how often, how long it lasts, who comes first, and how many orgasms you have. Instead, I want to address the questions that don't have easy answers. This book speaks about eroticism and the poetics of sex, the nature of erotic desire and its attendant dilemmas. When you love someone, how does it feel? And when you desire someone, how is it different? Does good intimacy always lead to good sex? Why is it that the transition to parenthood so often spells erotic disaster? Why is the forbidden so erotic? Is it possible to want what we already have?

We all share a fundamental need for security, which propels us toward committed relationships in the first place; but we have an equally strong need for adventure and excitement. Modern romance promises that it's possible to meet these two distinct sets of needs in one place. Still, I'm not convinced. Today, we turn to one person to provide what an entire village once did: a sense of grounding, meaning, and continuity. At the same time, we expect our committed relationships to be romantic as well as emotionally and sexually fulfilling. Is it any wonder that so many relationships crumble under the weight of it all? It's hard to generate excitement, anticipation, and lust with the same person you look to for comfort and stability, but it's not impossible. I invite you to think about ways you might introduce risk to safety, mystery to the familiar, and novelty to the enduring.

On the way, we will address how the modern ideology of love sometimes collides with the forces of desire. Love flourishes in an atmosphere of closeness, mutuality, and equality. We seek to know our beloved, to keep him near, to contract the distance between us. We care about those we love, worry about them, and feel responsible for them. For some of us, love and desire are inseparable. But for many others, emotional intimacy inhibits erotic expression. The caring, protective elements that foster love often block the unselfconsciousness that fuels erotic pleasure.

My belief, reinforced by twenty years of practice, is that in the course of establishing security, many couples confuse love with merging. This mix-up is a bad omen for sex. To sustain an élan toward the other, there must be a synapse to cross. Eroticism requires separateness. In other words, eroticism thrives in the space between the self and the other. In order to commune with the one we love, we must be able to tolerate this void and its pall of uncertainties.

With this paradox to chew on, consider another: desire is often accompanied by feelings that would seem to cramp love's style. Aggression, jealousy, and discord come to mind, for starters. I will explore the cultural pressures that shape domesticated sex, making it fair, equal, and safe, but also producing many bored couples. I'd like to suggest that we might have more exciting, playful, even frivolous sex if we were less constrained by our cultural penchant for democracy in the bedroom.

To buttress this notion, I take the reader on a detour into social history. We'll see that contemporary couples invest more in love than ever before; yet, in a cruel twist of fate it is this very model of love and marriage that is behind the exponential rise in the divorce rate. Here it behooves us to question whether traditional marital structures can ever meet the modern mandate, especially when "till death do us part" entails a life span double that of past centuries.

The magic elixir that's meant to make this possible is intimacy. We'll get to the bottom of this by looking through various lenses, but here it's worth pointing out that the stereotype of women as entirely romantic and men as sexual conquistadors should have been dispelled a long time ago. The same goes for any ideas that cast women as longing for love, essentially faithful, and domestically inclined, and men as biologically non-monogamous and fearful of intimacy. As a result of social and economic changes that have occurred in recent western history, traditional gender lines have been circumvented, and these qualities are now seen in both men and women. While stereotypes can hold considerable truth, they fall short of capturing the complexities of contemporary relationships. I seek a more androgynous approach to love.

As a couples therapist, I have inverted the usual therapeutic priorities. In my field we are taught to inquire about the state of the union first and then ask how this is manifested in the bedroom. Seen this way, the sexual relationship is a metaphor for the overall relationship. The underlying assumption is that if we can improve the relationship, the sex will follow. But in my experience, this is often not the case.

Traditionally, the therapeutic culture has favored the spoken word over the expressiveness of the body. Yet sexuality and emotional intimacy are two separate languages. I would like to restore the body to its rightful prominent place in discussions about couples and eroticism. The body often contains emotional truths that words can too easily gloss over. The very dynamics that are a source of conflict in a relationship—particularly those pertaining to power, control, dependency, and vulnerability—often become desirable when experienced through the body and eroticized. Sex becomes both a way to illuminate conflicts and confusion around intimacy and desire and a way to begin to heal these destructive splits. Each partner's body, imprinted as it is with the individual's history and the culture's admonitions, becomes a text to be read by all of us together.

In keeping with the theme of reading, this is as good a time as any to explain some terms you'll encounter in this book. For clarity,

I will use the word "marriage" to refer to long-term emotional commitments, not just to a legal status. And I sometimes like to move freely between male and female pronouns without necessarily heaping judgment on either gender.

I myself, as my name gives away, am of the female persuasion. Less obvious, perhaps, is that I'm a cultural hybrid. I live on many shores, and I want to bring an informed cultural view—or multicultural view—to the topic of this book. I grew up in Belgium, studied in Israel, and finished my training in the United States. Shuttling between various cultures for more than thirty years, I have formed the perspective of someone who is comfortable watching from the sidelines. This vantage point has provided me with multiple perspectives for my observations on how we develop sexually, how we connect to one another, how we narrate love, and how we engage in the pleasures of the body.

I've transferred my personal experience to my professional work as a clinician, teacher, and consultant working in cross-cultural psychology. Having focused on cultural transition, I've specifically worked with three populations: refugee families and international families (the two groups that move most these days, albeit for very different reasons) and intercultural couples (which include interracial and interfaith pairings). For intercultural couples, the cultural shifts do not stem from a geographic move, but instead take place in their own living rooms. What really piqued my interest was how this merging of cultures influenced gender relations and child-rearing practices. I pondered the many meanings of marriage, and how its role and its place in the larger family system varies in different national contexts. Is it a private act of two individuals or a communal affair between two families? In my sessions with couples, I tried to discern the cultural nuances behind the discussion of commitment, intimacy, pleasure, orgasm, and the body. Love may be universal, but its constructions in each culture are defined, both literally and figuratively, in different languages. I was particularly sensitive to the conversations about child and adolescent sexuality because it is in messages to children that societies most reveals their values, goals, incentives, prohibitions.

I speak eight languages. Some I learned at home, some at school, a few during my travels, and one or two through love. In my practice, I am called on to use my multicultural proficiency as well as my skill as a polyglot. My patients are straight and gay (I don't work with the transgender population at this time), married, committed, single, and remarried. They are young, old, and in between. They cover a wide spectrum of cultures, race, and class. Their individual stories highlight the cultural and psychological forces that shape how we love and how we desire.

One of my most formative personal experiences underlying this book may seem circuitous, but I must reveal it to you, as it sheds a light on the deeper motivations that fuel my passion. My parents were survivors of Nazi concentration camps. For a number of years, they stood face-to-face with death every day. My mother and father were the sole survivors of their respective families. They came out of this experience wanting to charge at life with a vengeance and to make the most of each day. They both felt that they had been granted a unique gift: living life again. My parents were unusual, I think. They didn't just want to survive; they wanted to revive. They possessed a thirst for life, thrived on exuberant experiences, and loved to have a good time. They cultivated pleasure. I know absolutely nothing about their sexual life except that they had two children, my brother and me. But by the way they lived, I sensed that they had a deep understanding of eroticism. Though I doubt that they ever used this word, they embodied its mystical meaning as a quality of aliveness, a pathway to freedom—not just the narrow definition of sex that modernity has assigned to it. It is this expanded understanding that I bring to bear on my discussion of eroticism in this book.

There is yet another powerful influence that has helped shape this project. My husband is the director of the International Trauma Studies Program at Columbia University. His work is devoted to assisting refugees, children of war, and victims of torture as they seek to overcome the massive trauma they've experienced. By restoring their sense of creativity and their capacity for play and pleasure, these survivors are ultimately helped to reconnect with life and the hope that fuels it. My husband deals with pain; I deal with pleasure. They are intimately acquainted.

The individuals I write about do not appear in the acknowledgments, though I owe them a great deal. Their stories are authentic and almost verbatim, but their identities are masked. Throughout this project, I've shared excerpts with them in the spirit of collaboration. Many of my ideas were developed through my work, and not the other way around. My ideas also draw on the wealth of careful considerations made by many professionals and authors who have previously tackled the ambiguities of love and desire.

Every day in my work I am confronted with the detailed realities that hide behind statistics. I see people who are such good friends that they cannot sustain being lovers. I see lovers who hold so tenaciously to the idea that sex must be spontaneous that they never have it at all. I see couples who view seduction as too much work, something they shouldn't have to do now that they're committed. I see others who believe that intimacy means knowing everything about each other. They abdicate any sense of separateness, then are left wondering where the mystery has gone. I see wives who would rather carry the label "low sexual desire" for the rest of their lives than suffer explaining to their husbands that foreplay needs to be more than a prelude to the real thing. I see people so desperate to beat back a feeling of deadness in their partnerships that they're willing to risk everything for a few moments of forbidden excitement with someone else. I see couples whose sex lives are rekindled by an affair, and others for whom an affair effectively ends what little connection remained. I see older men who feel betrayed by their newly unresponsive penises, who rush for Viagra to soften the anxiety of the hard facts; I see their wives made uncomfortable by the sudden challenge to their own passivity. I see new parents whose erotic energy has been sapped by caring for an infant—so consumed by their child that they don't remember to close the bedroom door once in a while. I see the man who looks at porn online not because he doesn't find his wife attractive but because her lack of enthusiasm leaves him feeling that there's something wrong with him for wanting sex. I see people so ashamed of their sexuality that they spare the one they love the ordeal. I see people who know they are loved, but who long to be desired. They all come to see me because they yearn for erotic vitality. Sometimes they come sheepishly; sometimes they arrive desperate, dejected, enraged. They don't just miss sex, the act; they miss the feeling of connection, playfulness, and renewal that sex allows them. I invite you to join me in my conversations with these questers as we work toward opening up and coming a step closer to transcendence.

For those who aspire to accelerate their heartbeat periodically, I give them the score: excitement is interwoven with uncertainty, and with our willingness to embrace the unknown rather than to shield ourselves from it. But this very tension leaves us feeling vulnerable. I caution my patients that there is no such thing as "safe sex."

I should point out, however, that not all lovers seek passion, or even, at one time, basked in it. Some relationships originate in feelings of warmth, tenderness, and nurturance, and the partners choose to remain in these calmer waters. They prefer a love that is built on patience more than on passion. To them, finding serenity in a lasting bond is what counts. There is no one way, and there is no right way.

Mating in Captivity aspires to engage you in an honest, enlightened, and provocative discussion. It encourages you to question yourself, to speak the unspoken, and to be unafraid to challenge sexual and emotional correctness. By flinging the doors open on erotic life and domesticity, I invite you to put the X back in sex.

Mating In
Captivity

From Adventure to Captivity

Why the Quest for Security Saps Erotic Vitality

> The original primordial fire of eroticism is sexuality; it raises the red flame of eroticism, which in turn raises and feeds another flame, tremulous and blue. It is the flame of love and eroticism. The double flame of life.
>
> —*Octavio Paz,* The Double Flame

PARTIES IN NEW YORK CITY are like anthropological field trips—you never know whom you'll meet or what you'll find. Recently I was milling around a self-consciously hip event, and, as is typical in this city of high achievers, before being asked my name I was asked what I do. I answered, "I'm a therapist, and I'm writing a book." The handsome young man standing next to me was also working on a book. "What are you writing about?" I asked him. "Physics," he answered. Politely, I mustered the next question, "What kind of physics?" I can't remember what his answer was, because the conversation about physics ended abruptly when someone asked me, "And you? What's your book about?" "Couples and eroticism," I answered.

Never was my Q rating as high—at parties, in cabs, at the nail salon, on airplanes, with teenagers, with my husband, you name it—as when I began writing a book about sex. I realize that there are certain topics that chase people away and others that act like magnets. People talk to me. Of course, that doesn't mean they tell me the truth. If there's one topic that invites concealment, it's this one.

"What about couples and eroticism?" someone asks.

"I'm writing about the nature of sexual desire," I reply. "I want to know if it's possible to keep desire alive in a long-term relationship, to avoid its usual wear."

"You don't necessarily need love for sex, but you need sex in love," says a man who's been standing on the sidelines, still undecided about which conversation to join.

"You focus mainly on married couples? Straight couples?" another asks. Read: is this book also about me? I reassure him, "I'm looking at myriad couples. Straight, gay, young, old, committed, and undecided."

I tell them I want to know how, or if, we can hold on to a sense of aliveness and excitement in our relationships. Is there something inherent in commitment that deadens desire? Can we ever maintain security without succumbing to monotony? I wonder if we can preserve a sense of the poetic, of what Octavio Paz calls the double flame of love and eroticism.

I've had this conversation many times, and the comments I heard at this party were hardly novel.

"Can't be done."

"Well, that's the whole problem of monogamy, isn't it?"

"That's why I don't commit. It has nothing to do with fear. I just hate boring sex."

"Desire over time? What about desire for one night?"

"Relationships evolve. Passion turns into something else."

"I gave up on passion when I had kids."

"Look, there are men you sleep with and men you marry."

As often happens in a public discussion, the most complex issues tend to polarize in a flash, and nuance is replaced with caricature. Hence the division between the romantics and the realists. The romantics refuse a life without passion; they swear that they'll never give up on true love. They are the perennial seekers, looking for the person with whom desire will never fizzle. Every time desire does wane, they conclude that love is gone. If eros is in decline, love must be on its deathbed. They mourn the loss of excitement and fear settling down.

At the opposite extreme are the realists. They say that enduring love is more important than hot sex, and that passion makes people do stupid things. It's dangerous, it creates havoc, and it's a weak foundation for marriage. In the immortal words of Marge Simpson, "Passion is for teenagers and foreigners." For the realists, maturity prevails. The initial excitement grows into something else—deep love, mutual respect, shared history, and companionship. Diminishing desire is inescapable. You are expected to tough it out and grow up.

As the conversation unfolds, the two camps eye each other with a complex alloy of pity, tenderness, envy, exasperation, and outright scorn. But while they position themselves at opposite ends of the spectrum, both agree with the fundamental premise that passion cools over time.

"Some of you resist the loss of intensity, some of you accept it, but all of you seem to believe that desire fades. What you disagree on is just how important the loss really is," I comment. Romantics value intensity over stability. Realists value security over passion. But both are often disappointed, for few people can live happily at either extreme.

Invariably, I'm asked if my book offers a solution. What can people do? Hidden behind this question looms a secret longing for the élan vital, the surge of erotic energy that marks our aliveness.

Whatever safety and security people have persuaded themselves to settle for, they still very much want this force in their lives. So I've become acutely attuned to the moment when all these ruminations about the inevitable loss of passion turn into expressions of hope. The real questions are these: Can we have both love and desire in the same relationship over time? How? What exactly would that kind of relationship be?

The Anchor and the Wave

Call me an idealist, but I believe that love and desire are not mutually exclusive, they just don't always take place at the same time. In fact, security and passion are two separate, fundamental human needs that spring from different motives and tend to pull us in different directions. In his book *Can Love Last?* the infinitely thoughtful psychoanalyst Stephen Mitchell offers a framework for thinking about this conundrum. As he explains it, we all need security: permanence, reliability, stability, and continuity. These rooting, nesting instincts ground us in our human experience. But we also have a need for novelty and change, generative forces that give life fullness and vibrancy. Here risk and adventure loom large. We're walking contradictions, seeking safety and predictability on one hand and thriving on diversity on the other.

Ever watch a child run away to explore and then run right back to make sure that Mom and Dad are still there? Little Sammy needs to feel secure in order to go into the world and discover; and once he has satisfied his need for exploration, he wants to go back to his safe base to reconnect. It's a sport he'll come back to as an adult, culminating in the games of eros. Periods of being bold and taking risks will alternate with periods of seeking grounding and safety. He may fluctuate, though he'll generally settle on one preference over another.

And what is true for human beings is true for every living thing: all organisms require alternating periods of growth and equilibrium. Any person or system exposed to ceaseless novelty and change risks falling into chaos; but one that is too rigid or static ceases to grow and eventually dies. This never-ending dance between change and stability is like the anchor and the waves.

Adult relationships mirror these dynamics all too well. We seek a steady, reliable anchor in our partner. Yet at the same time we expect love to offer a transcendent experience that will allow us to soar beyond our ordinary lives. The challenge for modern couples lies in reconciling the need for what's safe and predictable with the wish to pursue what's exciting, mysterious, and awe-inspiring.

For a lucky few, this is barely a challenge. These couples can easily integrate cleaning the garage with rubbing each other's back. For them, there is no dissonance between commitment and excitement, responsibility and playfulness. They can buy a home and be naughty in it, too. They can be parents and still be lovers. In short, they're able to seamlessly meld the ordinary and the uncanny. But for the rest of us, seeking excitement in the same relationship in which we establish permanence is a tall order. Unfortunately, too many love stories develop in such a way that we sacrifice passion so as to achieve stability.

So What Is It I Want?

Adele comes into my office holding half a sandwich in one hand and some paperwork she's doing on the fly in the other. At thirty-eight, she is a well-established lawyer in private practice. She's been married to Alan for seven years. It is a second marriage for both of them, and they have a daughter, Emilia, who's five. Adele is dressed simply and elegantly, though she's been meaning to get to the hairdresser for a while now and it shows.

"I want to get right to it," she says. "Eighty percent of the time I'm happy with him. I'm really happy." Not a minute to waste for this organized and accomplished woman. "He doesn't say certain things; he doesn't gush; but he's a really nice guy. I pick up the newspaper, and I feel fortunate. We're all healthy; we have enough money; our house has never caught on fire; we don't have to dodge bullets on the way home from work. I know how bad it can be out there. So what is it I want?

"I look at my friend Marc, who's getting divorced from his third wife because, he says, 'She doesn't inspire me.' So I ask Alan, 'Do I inspire you?' and you know what he says? 'You inspire me to cook chicken every Sunday.' He makes a fantastic coq au vin and you know why? Because he wants to please me; he knows I like it.

"So I'm trying to figure out what it is that I miss. You know that feeling you have the first year, that fluttery, exciting feeling, the butterflies in your stomach, the physical passion? I don't even know if I can get that anymore. And when I bring this up to Alan, he gets this face. 'Oh, you want to talk about Brad and Jen again?' Even Brad Pitt and Jennifer Aniston got tired of each other, right? I've studied biology; I know how the synapses work, how overuse lessens the reaction; I get that. Excitement wanes, yeah yeah yeah. But even if I can't have that fluttery butterfly feeling, I want to feel something.

"The realistic part of me knows that the excitement in the beginning is because of the insecurity in not quite knowing what he's feeling. When we were dating and the phone rang the reason it was exciting was that I didn't know it would be him. Now when he travels I tell him *not* to call me. I don't want to be woken up. The more intelligent part of me says, 'I don't want insecurity. I'm married. I have a kid. I don't need to worry every time he leaves town: Does he like me? Does he not like me? Is he going to cheat?'

You know those magazine tests: How to tell if he really loves you. I don't want to worry about that. I don't need that with my husband right now. But I'd like to recapture some of that excitement.

"By the end of a long day at work, taking care of Emilia and cooking a meal, cleaning up, checking things off my list, sex is the farthest thing from my mind. I don't even want to talk to anyone. Sometimes Alan watches TV and I go into the bedroom to read and I am very happy. So what is it I'm trying to put into words here? Because I'm not just talking about sex. I want to be appreciated *as a woman*. Not as a mother, not as a wife, not as a companion. And I want to appreciate him *as a man*. It could be a gaze, a touch, a word. I want to be looked at without all the baggage.

"He says it goes both ways. He's right. It's not like I put on my negligee and go hubba hubba. I'm lazy in the 'make me feel special' department. When we first met I bought him a briefcase for his birthday—something he saw in a store window and loved—and it had two tickets to Paris inside. This year I gave him a DVD and we celebrated with a couple of friends by eating a meat loaf his mother had made. Nothing against meat loaf, but that's what it's come to. I don't know why I don't do more. I've become complacent."

Adele, in her breathless riff, vividly captures the tension between the comfort of committed love and its muting effect on erotic vitality. Familiarity is indeed reassuring, and it brings a sense of security that Adele would never dream of giving up. At the same time, she wants to recapture the quality of aliveness and excitement that she and Alan had in the beginning. She wants both the coziness and the edge, and she wants them both with him.

The Era of Pleasure

Not so long ago, the desire to feel passionate about one's husband would have been considered a contradiction in terms. Historically, these two realms of life were organized separately—marriage on one side and passion most likely somewhere else, if anywhere at all. The concept of romantic love, which came about toward the end of the nineteenth century, brought them together for the first time. The central place of sex in marriage, and the heightened expectations surrounding it, took decades more to arrive.

The social and cultural transformations of the past fifty years have redefined modern coupledom. Alan and Adele are beneficiaries of the sexual revolution of the 1960s, women's liberation, the availability of birth control pills, and the emergence of the gay movement. With the widespread use of the pill, sex became liberated from reproduction. Feminism and gay pride fought to define sexual expression as an inalienable right. Anthony Giddens describes this transition in *The Transformation of Intimacy* when he explains that sexuality became a property of the self, one that we develop, define, and renegotiate throughout our lives. Today, our sexuality is an open-ended personal project; it is part of who we are, an identity, and no longer merely something we do. It has become a central feature of intimate relationships, and sexual satisfaction, we believe, is our due. The era of pleasure has arrived.

These developments, in conjunction with postwar economic prosperity, have contributed to a period of unmatched freedom and individualism. People today are encouraged to pursue personal fulfillment and sexual gratification, and to break free of the constraints of a social and family life heretofore defined by duty and obligation. But trailing in the shadow of this manifest extravagance lies a new kind of gnawing insecurity. The extended family, the community, and religion may indeed have limited our freedom, sexual and otherwise, but in return they offered us a much-needed sense of belonging. For generations, these traditional institutions provided order, meaning, continuity, and social support. Dismantling them has left us with more choices and fewer restrictions than ever. We are freer, but also more alone. As Giddens describes it, we have become ontologically more anxious.

We bring to our love relationships this free-floating anxiety. Love, beyond providing emotional sustenance, compassion, and companionship, is now expected to act as a panacea for existential aloneness as well. We look to our partner as a bulwark against the vicissitudes of modern life. It is not that our human insecurity is greater today than in earlier times. In fact, quite the contrary may be true. What is different is that modern life has deprived us of our traditional resources, and has created a situation in which we turn to one person for the protection and emotional connections that a multitude of social networks used to provide. Adult intimacy has become overburdened with expectations.

Of course, when Adele describes the state of her marriage she isn't thinking about contemporary angst. But I believe that the perils of love are heightened by the particular modern pangs we bring to it. We live miles away from our families, no longer know our childhood friends, and are regularly uprooted and transplanted. All this discontinuity has a cumulative effect. We bring to our romantic relationships an almost unbearable existential vulnerability—as if love itself weren't dangerous enough.

A Modern Love Story: The Short Version

You meet someone through a potent alchemy of attraction. It is a sweet reaction and it's always a surprise. You're filled with a sense of possibility, of hope, of being lifted out of the mundane and into a world of emotion and enthrallment. Love grabs you, and you feel powerful. You cherish the rush, and you want to hold on to the feeling. You're also scared. The more you become attached, the more you have to lose. So you set out to make love more secure. You seek to fix it, to make it dependable. You make your first commitments, and happily give up a little bit of freedom in exchange for a little bit of stability. You create comfort through devices—habit, ritual, pet names—that bring reassurance. But the excitement was bound to a certain measure of insecurity. Your high resulted from the uncertainty, and now, by seeking to harness it, you wind up draining the vitality out of the relationship. You enjoy the comfort, but complain that you feel constrained. You miss the spontaneity. In your attempt to control the risks of passion, you have tamed it out of existence. Marital boredom is born.

While love promises us relief from aloneness, it also heightens our dependence on one person. It is inherently vulnerable. We tend to assuage our anxieties through control. We feel safer if we can contract the distance between us, maximize the certainty, minimize the threats, and contain the unknown. Yet some of us defend against the uncertainties of love with such zeal that we cut ourselves off from its richness.

There's a powerful tendency in long-term relationships to favor the predictable over the unpredictable. Yet eroticism thrives on the unpredictable. Desire butts heads with habit and repetition. It is unruly, and it defies our attempts at control. So where does that leave us? We don't want to throw away the security, because our relationship depends on it. A sense of physical and emotional safety is basic to healthy pleasure and connection. Yet without an element of uncertainty there is no longing, no anticipation, no frisson. The motivational expert Anthony Robbins put it succinctly when he explained that passion in a relationship is commensurate with the amount of uncertainty you can tolerate.

Having New Eyes

How are we to introduce this uncertainty into our intimate relationships? How are we to create this gentle imbalance? In truth, it is already there. Eastern philosophers have long known that imper-manence is the only constant. Given the transient nature of life, given its ceaseless flux, there is more than a hint of arrogance in the assumption that we can make our relationships permanent, and that security can actually be fixed. As the adage says: "If you want to make God laugh, tell him your plans." Yet with blind faith we forge ahead. As loyal citizens of the modern world we believe in our own efficacy.

We liken the passion of the beginning to adolescent intoxica-tion—both transient and unrealistic. The consolation for giving it up is the security that waits on the other side. Yet when we trade passion for stability, are we not merely swapping one fantasy for another? As Stephen Mitchell points out, the fantasy of perma-nence may trump the fantasy of passion, but both are products of our imagination. We long for constancy, we may labor for it, but it is never guaranteed. When we love we always risk the possibility of loss—by criticism, rejection, separation, and ultimately death—regardless of how hard we try to defend against it. Introducing uncertainty sometimes requires nothing more than letting go of the illusion of certitude. In this shift of perception, we recognize the inherent mystery of our partner.

I point out to Adele that if we are to maintain desire with one person over time we must be able to bring a sense of unknown into a familiar space. In the words of Proust, "The real voyage of discovery consists not in seeking new landscapes but in having new eyes."

Adele recalls a moment when she experienced just this kind of perceptual shift. "Let me tell you what happened two weeks ago," she says. "It is so rare that I even remember the moment. We were at a work function, and Alan was talking with some colleagues, and I looked at him and thought: he's so attractive. It was almost weird, like an out-of-body experience. And you know what was so attractive? For a moment there I forgot that he's my husband and a real pain in the ass, obnoxious, stubborn, that he annoys me, that he leaves his mess all over the floor. At that moment I saw him as if I didn't know all that, and I was drawn to him like in the beginning. He's very smart; he talks well; he has this soothing, sexy way about him. I wasn't thinking about all our stupid exchanges when we bicker in the morning because I'm running late, or why did you do this, or what's going on for Christmas, or we have to talk about your mother. I was away from all that inane stuff and those absurd conversations. I just really saw him. That's how I felt, and I wonder if he ever feels like that about me anymore."

When I ask Adele if she has ever told Alan of that experience, she is quick to let me know that she hasn't. "No way. He'll make fun of me." I suggest that maybe the waning of romance is less about the bounds of familiarity and the weight of reality than it is about fear. Eroticism is risky. People are afraid to allow themselves these moments of idealization and yearning for the person they live with. It introduces a recognition of the other's sovereignty that can feel destabilizing. When our partner stands alone, with his own will and freedom, the delicateness of our bond is magnified. Adele's vulnerability is obvious in the way she wonders if Alan ever feels this way about her.

The typical defense against this threat is to stay within the realm of the familiar and the affectionate—the trivial bickering, the comfortable sex, the quotidian aspects of life that keep us tethered to reality and bar any chance of transcendence.

But when Adele looks at Alan out of the context of their marriage—switching from a zoom lens to a wide-angle—his otherness is accentuated, and that in turn heightens Adele's attraction to him. She sees him *as a man*. She has transformed someone familiar into someone still unknown after all these years.

Just When You Thought You Knew Her . . .

If uncertainty is a built-in feature of all relationships, so too is mystery. Many of the couples who come to therapy imagine that they know everything there is to know about their mate. "My husband doesn't like to talk." "My girlfriend would never flirt with another man. She's not the type." "My lover doesn't do therapy." "Why don't you just say it? I know what you're thinking?" "I don't need to give her lavish presents; she knows I love her." I try to highlight for them how little they've seen, urging them to recover their curiosity and catch a glimpse behind the walls that barricade the other.

In truth, we never know our partner as well as we think we do. Mitchell reminds us that even in the dullest marriages, predictability is a mirage. Our need for constancy limits how much we are willing to know the person who's next to us. We are invested in having him or her conform to an image that is often a creation of our own imagination, based on our own set of needs. "One thing about him is that he's never anxious. He's like a rock. I'm so neurotic." "He's too much of a wimp to leave me." "She doesn't put up with any of my shit." "We're both very traditional. Even though she has a PhD, she really likes staying home with the kids." We see what we want to see, what we can tolerate seeing, and our partner does the same. Neutralizing each other's complexity affords us a kind of manageable otherness. We narrow down our partner, ignoring or rejecting essential parts when they threaten the established order of our coupledom. We also reduce ourselves, jettisoning large chunks of our personalities in the name of love.

Yet when we peg ourselves and our partners to fixed entities, we needn't be surprised that passion goes out the window. And I'm sorry to say that the loss is on both sides. Not only have you squeezed out the passion, but you haven't really gained safety, either.

The fragility of this manufactured equilibrium becomes obvious when one partner breaks the rules of the contrivance and insists on bringing more authentic parts of himself into the relationship.

This is what happened to Charles and Rose. Married for almost four decades, they've had a lot of time to define one another. Charles is mercurial, a provocateur, and a playful seducer. He is a passionate man in need of a container, someone to help him channel the unbridled energies that distract him. "If it weren't for Rose, I don't think I would have the career and family I have today," he says. Rose is strong, independent, and clearheaded. She possesses a kind of natural equanimity that calibrates his intemperateness. As they describe it, she is the solid; he, the fluid. The few times Rose ventured into passionate territory before meeting Charles, she found it overwhelming. It left her depleted and unhappy. What he represents for her is passion that she doesn't have to own. What scares Rose is the loss of control and what scares Charles is that he enjoys the loss of control too much. The complementarity of their relationship allows them to flourish within a bounded space.

This fertile arrangement worked reasonably well until the day it didn't. As so often happens, there is a moment when we recognize that what we're doing is no longer working. Often it follows significant events that make us review the meaning and the structure of our lives. Suddenly, the compromises that worked so well yesterday become sacrifices we no longer want to brook today. For Charles, a succession of losses—the death of his mother, the death of a close friend, and a scare regarding his own health—have made him keenly aware of his own mortality. He wants to charge at life, to ply his vitality, to reconnect with the exuberance that he's kept in check in order to be with Rose. He can no longer bear to keep that part of himself tucked away, even in exchange for the solid ground Rose offers. But every time he tries to talk about this hunger, Rose feels threatened and dismisses him. "You're having another midlife crisis? What are you going to do, buy a red Trans-Am?"

Rose and Charles have both had their nonmonogamous interludes over the years. The facts were known, the details were not; and they put these episodes behind them. Or at least Rose did. "I thought we were past our turbulent years. We're in our sixties, for God's sake," she moans.

"And that precludes what?" I ask her.

"Hurting me! Risking our marriage! I've come to accept the terms of our relationship. Why can't he?"

"And those terms are?"

"When we married, we loved each other very much. We still do. But, shall we say, we had both known stronger passions. Charles came out of it disillusioned—the high intensity was always short-lived, and he was left with women he didn't have much in common with. I came out of it relieved. I got too lost in it. We talked about it back then, that we were both looking for something more enduring and a little calmer." Rose goes on to explain that she and Charles had other goals for their marriage—companionship, intellectual stimulation, physical and emotional care, support. "We really valued what we had found with each other."

Rose grew up poor. Her father ran a junkyard in rural Tennessee. Today she has a corner office on the fifty-sixth floor overlooking Madison Avenue in Manhattan. "My hillbilly town wasn't exactly supportive of girls with ambition, and I had a lot. When I met Charles, I knew he was different. I could be with him and he would let me do my own thing. In the early 1960s, that was a big deal."

"What did you think was going to happen sexually? That was a big deal in the sixties, too," I say.

"I was OK with our sex life. I thought it was fine, even nice," she tells me. "I've always known that for Charles it wasn't enough, but I expected him to deal with it."

In a private session with Charles a few weeks later, Charles gives me his take on things. "Sex with Rose is nice, but it's always been kind of flat. Sometimes I can deal with the low intensity; other times it's been unbearable. I've gone online, I've gone outside of the marriage, I've gone to Rose. Mostly I tried to squelch it, because there doesn't seem to be room for this between us. But I don't want to do that anymore. Life is too short. I'm getting older. When I feel erotically alive, as you call it, I don't worry about death and I don't worry about my age, at least for a few moments.

"Frankly, I'm surprised at her reaction," he continues. "It's been years since she was interested in sex. This may sound strange, but I honestly didn't think she'd feel so strongly about my being involved with other women. Even though I'm not exclusive any longer, I'm as emotionally faithful and committed as I've always been. I don't want to hurt her, and I certainly don't want to leave her, but something had to change for me."

Charles isn't behaving according to the script, but then neither is Rose. She is fragile and afraid, not the invincible woman Charles needs her to be. Just as they had banished his seductiveness, they had also suppressed her vulnerability. They have outgrown their respective roles, and they are in a crisis.

Unbeknownst to them, this may be the greatest opportunity for expansion they've had in years, for it allows them to express parts of themselves that have long been denied. It's tiresome to have to be in control all the time, and Rose was due for a break. It's equally draining to feel erotically impoverished, and Charles's refusal to tolerate this situation was his first step in bringing more authentic parts of himself to Rose. Ironically, in the midst of this emotional turmoil they began making love again after many years apart. Rose's desire for Charles came back to life in tandem with his interest in other women. The more he eludes her, the more she wants him. And for his part, seeing her care so much about what he does has a profound erotic appeal.

For a long time their relationship operated on a contract of mutuality. They were not to express feelings or needs that exceeded what they had been allocated. They were not to be irrational, insensitive, or greedy. Now, however, they both were making strong claims. They made demands on each other that they didn't want to give up on. There was a lot of pain, but at the same time there was a vibrancy that neither could deny.

"I haven't felt this lousy in years," Rose tells me. "But underneath, I can see it needed to happen. I've always focused on the tangible stuff—the money, the house, the kids in college—thinking that's what's solid. But who says that what Charles is after is so frivolous? Maybe it's another way of taking care of a marriage."

By refusing to acknowledge anything that falls outside the accepted range of behavior, Charles and Rose had achieved the opposite of what they were seeking. Rather than making their love more secure, they had, in fact, made it more vulnerable. But allowing both of them to reveal heretofore segregated parts of themselves was not without risk. The very foundation of their relationship was at stake. Each of them would have to tolerate the unfolding of the other, even if it took them beyond their range of comfort.

Dismantling the Security System

We often expect our relationship to act as a buttress against the slings and arrows of life. But love, by its very nature, is unstable. So we shore it up: we tighten the borders, batten down the hatches, and create predictability, all in an effort to make us feel more secure. Yet the mechanisms that we put in place to make love safer often put us more at risk. We ground ourselves in familiarity, and perhaps achieve a peaceful domestic arrangement, but in the process we orchestrate boredom. The verve of the relationship collapses under the weight of all that control. Stultified, couples are left wondering, "Whatever happened to fun? What ever happened to excitement, to transcendence, to awe?"

Desire is fueled by the unknown, and for that reason it's inherently anxiety-producing. In his book *Open to Desire*, the Buddhist psychoanalyst Mark Epstein explains that our willingness to engage that mystery keeps desire alive. Faced with the irrefutable otherness of our partner, we can respond with fear or with curiosity. We can try to reduce the other to a knowable entity, or we can embrace her persistent mystery. When we resist the urge to control, when we keep ourselves open, we preserve the possibility of discovery. Eroticism resides in the ambiguous space between anxiety and fascination. We remain interested in our partners; they delight us, and we're drawn to them. But, for many of us, renouncing the illusion of safety, and accepting the reality of our fundamental insecurity, proves to be a difficult step.

2

More Intimacy, Less Sex
Love Seeks Closeness, but Desire Needs Distance

> Love and lust are inseparable parts of a larger whole for some, while for others they are irretrievably disconnected. Most of us, however, express our eroticism somewhere in the gray areas where love and lust both relate and conflict.
>
> —*Jack Morin, from* The Erotic Mind

IN ANY FIRST CONVERSATION WITH a couple, I always ask how they met and what attracted them to each other. Since we associate therapy with problems, people usually don't come to me when they are still in the initial thrall of love. Sometimes they need a gentle reminder of what once was. It can be difficult for estranged or distressed couples to focus on what drew them together, but within every couple's "creation myth" lies the key to understanding the unfolding story of their relationship.

"She was beautiful." "He was so smart and funny." "He had pizzazz, and he exuded such self-confidence and style." "For me it was her warmth." "For me it was his gentleness." "I knew she wouldn't leave me." "I loved his hands." "His dick." "Her eyes." "His voice." "He made great omelets." The attributes that describe an idealized lover are always luxurious and bountiful. Love is an exercise in selective perception, even a delicious deception as well, though who cares about that in the beginning?

We magnify the good qualities of those we love, and confer on them almost mythical powers. We transform them, and we in turn are transformed in their presence. "He made me laugh." "She made me feel special, smart." "We could talk for hours." "I knew I could trust her." "I felt so accepted." "He made me feel beautiful." Such comments highlight the magnificence of the beloved or illuminate his capacity to enlarge us, to lift us from ourselves. As the psychoanalyst Ethel Spector Person writes, "Love arises from within ourselves as an imaginative act, a creative synthesis that aims to fulfill our deepest longings, our oldest dreams, that allows us both to renew and transform ourselves." Love is at once an affirmation and a transcendence of who we are.

Beginnings are always ripe with possibilities, for they hold the promise of completion. Through love we imagine a new way of being. You see me as I've never seen myself. You airbrush my imperfections, and I like what you see. With you, and through you, I will become that which I long to be. I will become whole. Being chosen by the one you chose is one of the glories of falling in love. It generates a feeling of intense personal importance. I matter. You confirm my significance.

As I listen to couples describe the merging that accompanies the nascence of love, I get a glimpse of the dreams that propelled them toward each other. The first stage of any encounter is filled with fantasies. It's a stream of projections, anticipations, and stirrings that may or may not evolve into a relationship. Here you are in front of someone you barely know, and you imagine climbing Kilimanjaro together, building an *Architectural Digest* home, making babies, or umpteen irresistible fantasies as arbitrary as the weather. As my patients recount the exaltation they felt, I am able to take a peek beneath the rubble to see what they once had.

A Hopeful State of Bliss

John and Beatrice spent their first six months virtually locked up in a room in a blissful state of effervescence. John is a stockbroker who has known the glories and defeats of the dot-com revolution. When I first met him in therapy he had just witnessed his fortune wither before his eyes. He would spend days staring at his computer screen, helplessly tracking the demise of his portfolio while he drank the last of his single-malt Scotch. He had also just experienced an erotic collapse in the midst of an otherwise loving and caring relationship with a girlfriend of five years. He was in the grip of a triple crisis—emotional, professional, and financial. When he met Beatrice, it was like waking up from a coma. His sense of relief and renewal was profound. Beatrice, a Pre-Raphaelite beauty, was a graduate student in English in her mid-twenties, ten years younger than John. In the cocoon under the sheets they would talk for hours, make love, talk again, make love, and sleep (but very little). Transported as they were in this early rapture, they felt free and open. They relished the meeting of their two worlds, were endlessly curious, and luxuriated in their feelings of mutuality and warmth, free from the torments of the outside world.

As the relationship between them evolved, John and Beatrice experienced a growing sense of serenity. The initial excitement matured, the real world reemerged, and hope was transformed into substance. Enter intimacy. If love is an act of imagination, then intimacy is an act of fruition. It waits for the high to subside so it can patiently insert itself into the relationship. The seeds of intimacy are time and repetition. We choose each other again and again, and so create a community of two.

When they move in together, John and Beatrice are introduced to each other's tastes and preferences, and become more acquainted with each other's quirks. John likes his coffee black. No sugar. And he needs his first cup as soon as he gets out of bed. Beatrice likes hers with cream, no sugar, but she likes to have a glass of water first. Some of these wants are met with ease and tenderness; some they must learn to accept; and some are annoying, offensive, or downright disgusting. They wonder how they'll ever live with . . . (name the three most revolting habits of your own partner). They enter into each other's world of habit, and this familiarity reassures them. It creates routine, which in turn fosters a sense of security. Growing familiarity also signals freedom from ceremony and constraint. Yet this unceremoniousness, which is a welcome feature of intimacy, is a proven antiaphrodisiac as well.

Of course, familiarity is but one manifestation of intimacy. Our continued discovery of another person extends far beyond surface habits into an interior world of thoughts, beliefs, and feelings. We penetrate our partner mentally. We talk, we listen, we share, and we compare. We disclose certain parts of ourselves, while we adorn, fiddle with, and conceal others. Sometimes I learn something about you because you tell me: your history, your family, your life before we met. But just as often my understanding comes from watching you, intuiting, and making associations. You present the facts, I connect the dots, and an image is formed. Your singularities are gradually revealed to me, openly or covertly, intentionally or not. Some places inside of you are easy to reach; others are encrypted and laborious to decode. Over time, I come to know your values, and your fault lines. By witnessing how you move in the world, I come to know how you connect: what excites you, what presses your buttons, and what you're afraid of. I come to know your dreams and your nightmares. You grow on me. And all this, of course, happens in two directions.

As John settles into this new relationship, he stops talking about it in therapy, and I assume that no talk means no problems. So when, after a year, he brings it up again, I pay close attention.

"Things are going well. We've moved in together. We get along great. She's beautiful, she's funny, she's smart. I really love her. We don't have sex."

Intimacy Begets Sexuality . . . or Does It?

The prevailing belief of couples therapy in America today is that sex is a metaphor for the relationship—find out what's going on emotionally and you can infer what's going on in the bedroom. If couples are caring and nurturing—if they have good communication, mutual respect, fairness, trust, empathy, and honesty—you can reliably assume an ongoing, pulsing erotic bond. In her book *Hot Monogamy*, Dr. Patricia Love gives voice to these ideas:

> *Good verbal communication is one of the keys to a good sex life. When couples share their thoughts and emotions freely throughout the day, they create between them a high degree of trust and emotional connection, which gives them the freedom to explore their sexuality more fully. Intimacy begets sexuality.*

For many people, a loving, committed relationship is indeed a great enhancer of sexual desire, a fillip. They feel accepted and swaddled, and that safety allows them to feel free. The trust that comes with emotional closeness enables them to unleash their erotic appetites. But what about John and Beatrice? They don't fill the bill. They have a beautiful, intimate, loving relationship (they communicate); and, according to this view, that should form the basis for sustained desire. But it doesn't. And if it's any consolation to them, it doesn't work this way for a lot of people.

Ironically, what makes for good intimacy does not always make for good sex. It may be counterintuitive, but it's been my experience as a therapist that increased emotional intimacy is often accompanied by decreased sexual desire. This is indeed a puzzling inverse correlation: the breakdown of desire appears to be an unintentional consequence of the creation of intimacy. I can think of many couples whose opening lines in my office go something like this: "We really love each other. We have a good relationship. But we don't have sex." Joe relishes Rafael's intense interest in him but doesn't like being engulfed physically—Joe will only be a "top." Susan and Jenny feel closer than ever after they adopt their first child together, but that closeness does not translate into sensuality. Adele and Alan refer to their nights away at a hotel as intimate, but not particularly passionate. Despite their erotic frustrations, these couples seem to share a fine intimacy, not a lack thereof.

Andrew and Serena are clear that sex has been an issue from the beginning, and that regardless of how much their relationship has flourished, it is never enough to charge them erotically. Before she met Andrew, Serena had experienced a luscious sexual life in a number of long-term relationships. In her experience, mounting intimacy had consistently led to better sex, so she was surprised when it didn't work that way with Andrew. When I asked her why she stayed with him when from the first date she didn't feel desired by him, she answered, "I thought we'd work on it. That with love it would get better." "Sometimes it is the love that stands in the way," I explained, "so just the opposite happens."

Listening to these men and women has led me to rethink what I had long assumed about the correlation between intimacy and sexuality. Rather than looking at sex as an exclusive outgrowth of the emotional relationship, I've come to see it as a separate entity. Sexuality is more than a metaphor for the relationship—it stands on its own as a parallel narrative.

The intimate story of a couple can indeed tell us a lot about their erotic life, but it can't tell us everything. There is a complex relationship between love and desire, and it is not a cause-and-effect, linear arrangement. A couple's emotional life together and their physical life together each have their ebbs and flows, their ups and downs, but these don't always correspond. They intersect, they influence each other, but they're also distinct. That's one reason why, to the chagrin of many, you can often "fix" a relationship without doing anything for the sex. Maybe intimacy only sometimes begets sexuality.

Separateness Is a Precondition for Connection

It is too easily assumed that problems with sex are the result of a lack of closeness. But my point is that perhaps the way we construct closeness reduces the sense of freedom and autonomy needed for sexual pleasure. When intimacy collapses into fusion, it is not a lack of closeness but too much closeness that impedes desire.

Love rests on two pillars: surrender and autonomy. Our need for togetherness exists alongside our need for separateness. One does not exist without the other. With too much distance, there can be no connection. But too much merging eradicates the separateness of two distinct individuals. Then there is nothing more to transcend, no bridge to walk on, no one to visit on the other side, no other internal world to enter. When people become fused—when two become one—connection can no longer happen. There is no one to connect with. Thus separateness is a precondition for connection: this is the essential paradox of intimacy and sex.

The dual (and often conflicting) needs for connection and independence are a central theme in our developmental histories. Throughout childhood we struggle to find a delicate balance between our profound dependence on our primary caregivers and our need to carve out a sense of independence. The psychologist Michael Vincent Miller reminds us that this struggle is vividly represented in children's nightmares: "the abandonment dreams of falling or being lost, and the engulfment dreams of being attacked or devoured by monsters." We come to our adult relationships with an emotional memory box ready to be activated. The extent to which our childhood relationships nurture or obstruct both sets of needs will determine the vulnerabilities that we bring into our adult relationships—what we most want and what we most fear. We all straddle both needs. Their intensity and priority fluctuate throughout our lives; and, as it happens, we tend to choose partners whose proclivities match our vulnerabilities.

Some of us enter intimate bonds with an acute awareness of our need to connect, to be close, not to be alone, not to be abandoned. Others approach relationships with a heightened need for personal space—our sense of self-preservation inspires vigilance against being devoured. Erotic, emotional connection generates closeness that can become overwhelming, evoking claustrophobia. It can feel intrusive. What was initially a secure enclosure becomes confining. While our need for closeness is almost as basic as our need for food, it carries with it anxieties and threats that can inhibit desire. We want closeness, but not so much that we feel trapped by it.

All these meanderings on intimacy are still far from the awareness of John and Beatrice. The authenticity and the spontaneity of the beginning did not lead them to anticipate the ambivalence of love that would follow. From where they were, intimacy was simple. Open up, reveal, share, become transparent, open up more . . .

John and Beatrice exemplify a typical beginning. In fact, the intense physical and emotional fusion they experience is possible only with someone we don't yet know. At this early stage merging and surrendering are relatively safe, because the boundaries between the two people are still externally defined. John and Beatrice are new to each other. And while they are migrating into each other's respective worlds, they have not yet taken full residence; they are still two distinct entities. It is all the space between them that allows them to imagine no space at all. They are still enthralled by the encounter, and they have not yet consolidated their relationship.

In the beginning you can focus on the connection because the psychological distance is already there; it's a part of the structure. Otherness is a fact. You don't need to cultivate separateness in the early stages of falling in love; you still are separate. You aim to overcome that separateness. As new lovers, John and Beatrice enjoyed a built-in distance that allowed them to experience the confluence of love and desire freely, exempt from the conflicts they would bring to therapy later.

Entrapment Deadens Desire

For John, intimacy harbors a threat of entrapment. He grew up in a home with an alcoholic, abusive father. He can't remember a time when he wasn't acutely attuned to both his father's moods and his mother's sadness. As a young boy he was recruited to be his mother's emotional caretaker, and to alleviate her loneliness. He was her hope, her solace, a vicarious affirmation that her miserable life would be vindicated through her marvelous son. Children of such conflicted marriages are often enlisted to protect the vulnerable parent. John has never doubted his mother's deep love for him; nor has the love ever been without a sense of burden. From early on, love implied responsibility and obligation. And even while he craves the closeness of intimacy—he has always had a woman in his life—he doesn't know how to experience love in a way that does not feel confining. The emerging love he feels for Beatrice carries with it the same heaviness that love has always had for him.

There are many circumstances that can lead people to experience love and intimacy as constricting—an unhappy childhood is not a prerequisite. Popular love talk has made a real case for thinking of this as a "fear of intimacy," which is seen as afflicting men in particular. But what I observe is not so much a reluctance to engage in intimate bonding—no one can doubt John's deep involvement with Beatrice. Rather it is the weightiness of that involvement that these people find overbearing. Foreclosing the necessary freedom and spontaneity that eros demands, they feel trapped by intimacy.

John's sexual inhibitions are exacerbated as his emotional involvement with his girlfriend deepens. As a matter of fact, the more he cares about her, the less he can freely lust after her. For him, as for many other men in this predicament, erotic shutdown is not subtle. He is at the mercy of a stubborn penis that simply will not respond. But why? What is the erotic block that stops him from pursuing pleasure with Beatrice, the same woman with whom he lay in a langorous paradise not so long ago?

Ironically, even the closeness generated by good sex can have a boomerang effect. Like John and Beatrice, many couples experience their relationship as a dance in which great sex brings them close, but then this very closeness can make sex difficult again. The initial rapture facilitates a swift bonding and establishes an immediate connection. But while many of us relish the idea of losing ourselves in sex, the very oneness that we experience through the merging of our bodies can evoke a sense of obliteration. The intensity of sexual passion triggers a fear of engulfment. Of course, few of us are aware of these undercurrents as they're happening. What we feel instead is the urge to pull out right after orgasm, or the sudden desire to make a sandwich, to light a cigarette. We welcome the intrusion of any random thought: I meant to send an e-mail to . . . These windows need cleaning. . . . I wonder how my friend Jack is doing? We appreciate being left alone to meander leisurely in our own mind because this reestablishes a psychological distance, a delineation of the boundaries between me and you. From "inter-" we go back to "intra-." Having been all over each other, we retreat back into our own skin. Nowhere is the passage from connection to separateness represented more clearly than at the end of a sexual act.

In his book *Arousal*, the psychoanalyst Michael Bader offers another explanation for John and Beatrice's erotic impasse. In his view, intimacy comes with a growing concern for the well-being of the other person, which includes a fear of hurting her. But sexual excitement requires the capacity not to worry, and the pursuit of pleasure demands a degree of selfishness. Some people can't allow themselves this selfishness, because they're too absorbed with the well-being of the beloved. This emotional configuration is reminiscent of how John felt toward his mother—his awareness of her unhappiness overwhelmed him with worry and a sense of burden. The very caring he experiences makes it harder for him to focus on his own needs, to feel spontaneous, sexually alive, and carefree.

John has faced this vexing problem of loss of desire in every intimate relationship he's been in. In the past, every time the block set in he interpreted it as meaning that he no longer loved the woman. In fact, the contrary is true. It is because he loves her so much that he carries this sense of responsibility for her and can't enjoy the blithe quest for erotic rapture.

Patterns Are Equal Employment Opportunities

Dynamics in relationships are always complementary—both partners contribute to creating patterns. We can't talk about John's fear of entrapment and his diminishing desire without also taking a look at what Beatrice brings to the relationship. So I invite her to come in with John for a few sessions. In the course of our conversation her contribution to the puzzle becomes clear. In her coupling fervor, she has matched her interests to his, given up most activities that don't include him, and stopped seeing her friends. Unfortunately, all her attempts to increase the closeness between them have had the opposite effect erotically. Her eagerness to please and her constant readiness to give up anything that might come between them increases the emotional burden and further exacerbates his sexual withdrawal. It's as if his penis is creating a boundary that he cannot establish otherwise. It's hard to feel attracted to someone who has abandoned her sense of autonomy. Maybe he can love her, but it's clearly much harder for him to desire her. There's no tension.

I suggested that Beatrice move out of their joint living situation for a while, and reestablish some independence. Doing this encouraged her to reconnect with her friends and to stop organizing her life around John. As I said to her, "You're so afraid to lose him that you've alienated yourself and you've lost your freedom. There isn't a separate person here for him to love." To John I said, "You are such a caregiver that you can no longer be a lover. We need to reestablish a degree of differentiation and re-create some of the distance you had in the beginning. It's hard to experience desire when you're weighted down by concern."

In the next few months Beatrice did move out. In a remarkable turnaround she found her own apartment, sent in her application for a PhD program, took a trip with her friends, and started earning her own money. Gradually, as John became convinced that she had two feet to stand on, and as it became clear to Beatrice that she did not need to abdicate her own person to merit love, they created a space between them into which desire could flow more freely.

Many of the men and women I see in my practice find it particularly difficult to introduce this kind of emotional space into their loving relationships. You would think that the safety of an established base would make it easier to take these kinds of risks, but no. A secure relationship does indeed give us the courage to act on our professional ambitions, to confront family secrets, and to take the skydiving course we never dared consider before. Yet we balk at the idea of establishing distance within the relationship itself—the very place that grants us the delicious togetherness in the first place. We can tolerate space anywhere but there.

Sexual desire does not obey the laws that maintain peace and contentment between partners. Reason, understanding, compassion, and camaraderie are the handmaidens of a close, harmonious relationship. But sex often evokes unreasoning obsession rather than thoughtful judgment, and selfish desire rather than altruistic consideration. Aggression, objectification, and power all exist in the shadow of desire, components of passion that do not necessarily nurture intimacy. Desire operates along its own trajectory.

The Flannel Nightgown

My first meeting with Jimmy and Candace was a powerful illustration of this all too common story. Jimmy and Candace are young musicians in their early thirties who've been married for seven years. They are a biracial couple: she is African-American; he is of Irish descent. She exudes confidence in her boy jeans and aquamarine nails; he has the Quiksilver signature all over him. They're attractive, spunky, and on the go—and they are in despair over what's happening to them. "We're not having sex, and this has been going on for years," Candace explains. "We are terrified about it and so upset. And I think we each have a deep-rooted fear that we're going to find out it's unfixable."

Like John, Candace has experienced what feels like an inescapable loss of desire in every relationship she has been in; and what emerges from our conversation is that she understands her pattern. "My problem, my side of it, doesn't have to do with Jimmy," she explains. "When I'm intimate with someone, when I'm in love and he loves me, I suddenly lose interest sexually. I feel like there's something missing and I can't get close to my partner on a sexual level.

I had a number of long-term relationships before I met Jimmy, and it happened each time."

Candace knows who Jimmy is for her. He's reliable, thoughtful, and intelligent. They share a rich partnership. And while she wants these characteristics in a man, their collateral consequences are counter-erotic for her. Faced with Jimmy's kindness, she isn't able to experience her own sexual energy. "What I can tell you," she says, "is that his kindness makes me feel safe, but when I think about who I want to sleep with, safe is not what I look for."

"Because it's not what?" I ask her. "It's not transgressive enough? It's not aggressive enough?"

"It's not aggressive enough."

"And he is in some way too much of a conscientious lover?"

"Yeah."

"And he's constantly paying attention to you?"

"Which is very thoughtful."

"Very thoughtful indeed, but not exciting." I add. "It's all very affectionate, very cozy; it's just not sexual. You've replaced sensual love with something else. It's what the sex therapist Dagmar O'Connor calls comfort love."

Candace nods, "Like a flannel nightgown."

The caring, protective elements that nurture home life can go against the rebellious spirit of carnal love. We often choose a partner who makes us feel cherished; but after the initial romance we find, like Candace, that we can't sexualize him or her. We long to create closeness in our relationships, to bridge the space between our partner and ourselves, but, ironically, it is this very space between self and other that is the erotic synapse. In order to bring lust home, we need to re-create the distance that we worked so hard to bridge. Erotic intelligence is about creating distance, then bringing that space to life.

In one of our sessions Candace describes how nothing turns her on more than to see Jimmy perform onstage. But when I ask her if she ever goes backstage afterward, she tells me no. "Why don't you go into the dressing room?" I ask her. "You look at him up there onstage and you're all excited by him. He's totally in possession of himself and his talent. But then you wait until he comes home and he instantly becomes deeroticized." She nods in agreement; he looks disappointed.

"Why don't you divorce him?" I suggest. "Stay with him but divorce him. If you're not married to him, he won't look like such a homebody."

"You know what I said to him?" she admits, "I said, 'If you left me today I would be sexually interested in you.'"

Candace recognizes that the feeling of emotional closeness she longs for with Jimmy stands in the way of what excites her sexually. In order to circumvent this pitfall, she needs to create psychological distance. Long before meeting me, Candace had attempted to do just that. She had come up with her own solution to the predicament: Jimmy was to ignore her when he came home, rather than instantly approach her. As she said, "If I feel that you don't need me at all, you become desirable." Intuitively, without knowing why she needed this particular plot, she was trying to generate desire.

Unfortunately, Jimmy wasn't up for the game. He saw her need for being at arms-length as a rejection of him. He poignantly articulated his longing when he explained, "I've had so much anger. I remember a time when all I had to do was rub my knee up her thigh and she'd get all turned on. But for so long I haven't truly felt that she wanted me like that. I want her to want me. I want her to be hungry for one thing and one thing only. And that thing is me."

"Yet you see her request for a breather as rejection," I respond. "You know, desire acts in weird ways. Here she is asking you to ignore her, not to want her, as a way for her to want you. I can see why this makes no sense. Why such detours? And I understand your reaction. But you see, she needs to separate the intimate from the erotic, and for that she needs space. She invited you into a scheme that would allow her to do just that. It wasn't a rebuff; it was an invitation. You have to imagine it not literally, but as a form of sexual play. Play at not needing me. Play at ignoring me."

But Jimmy could not play, because he was caught in a struggle with Candace. He didn't want to engage in such contortions to elicit her desire. He wanted her to want him his way. Jimmy had felt deprived and rejected for so many years that the main feeling that escorted him was anger. His bile only highlighted the extent of his longing and need. The way they neutralized the threat of rage was through massive affection. Their almost constant physicality acted like a sexual appetite suppressor. This kind of contact can sustain itself for years without turning into desire. Unconditional love does not drive unconditional want. That's what we have with friends, and Jimmy and Candace were friends who wanted to be lovers.

Knowing that Candace had already expressed a need for distance, I saw an opening to intervene. I sought to introduce a disruption into the cozy, affectionate touch that had come to replace sex. "Do you touch each other?" I asked, though I already knew the answer.

"All the time," she replied.

"Do you cuddle?"

"Yes," Jimmy said.

"A lot?"

"Yes," they said in unison.

"Well, it's got to stop."

They looked at me wide-eyed. Here they had been emphasizing one aspect of their relationship that they both cherished, and I was taking it away from them. But by the way Candace responded, I knew I was on to something.

"You don't know what you're doing to me," she said. "I'm so touch-sensitive. For me, it's all about touch. I'll take it from anyone, even a relative stranger. I'm a touch whore." Jimmy added, "When we visited my family last week, my mother's best friend was rubbing her shoulders. You know, now that I think about it, I remember wondering if it even mattered whether it was me or Mrs. Monahan."

"So, this is going to be the goal of therapy," I interjected. "We're going to differentiate between Jimmy and Mrs. Monahan."

By telling them not to touch I was mapping a space that would give her room to go after him. That, in turn, would give him the feeling of being desired. "I'll make this clear for you. No contact. No pecks, no kissing, no massage, no strokes. Nothing. Sorry, you guys. You can write, you can send notes, you can make eyes—whatever else you want to do. Because at this point you have smothered sizzle with affection, leaving it with no way to ignite."

Candace was ready to comply with my suggestion. "OK," she agreed. "It's hateful, but it's a good idea."

I wondered who would have the harder time following my prescription. While Candace presented herself as the "touch whore," I suspected that Jimmy would be the first to break the agreement, for he had more at stake. He had been furious for years, and he had never known how to be angry with a person he also loves—how to be mad and connected at the same time. Behind his restraint, behind the sweet caresses, lay the unarticulated fear that ire inevitably leads to separation. During the first several weeks, Jimmy repeatedly slipped. So I instructed Candace to become more forceful in maintaining the hands-off rule. I was looking to up the ante. Eventually, Jimmy got worked up enough to comply. "About a month into it, I wanted nothing to do with her."

Removing the protective layer of affection turned out to be more effective than I had anticipated. "Safe might not be attractive to me," Candace admitted. "But I've come to rely on it. These last few weeks he's been more removed, and it's been really uncomfortable. We're not used to being this way. I got what I asked for, but I'm not sure it's what I wanted."

Candace and Jimmy had constructed an intimacy that precluded conflict of any sort. All the tension was crystallized in their sexual impasse. It was the one place where they maintained their distinction. By upsetting the balance of their harmonious but sexually flat relationship, I hoped to introduce an increased sense of otherness; for without that, there was no way desire would emerge.

A few months into our work together, Candace and Jimmy reported that they had noticed a difference, but they still had a long trek ahead. "In a lot of ways we have so much in terms of our relationship. We have a lot to be thankful for, and I know that," Candace told me. "But we've also come to realize that being close doesn't mean never fighting. It's funny, because the one thing that we were so proud of was actually kind of a problem."

In listening to Candace, it occurred to me that the word "safe" had more than one face. The psychologist Virginia Goldner makes an accurate distinction between the "flaccid safety of permanent coziness" and the "dynamic safety" of couples who fight and make up and whose relationship is a succession of breaches and repairs. It's not by co-opting aggression but rather by owning it that sexual tension can freely romp—and can itself bring safety.

Everyone Needs a Secret Garden

In her landmark book *The Second Sex*, Simone de Beauvoir writes, "Eroticism is a movement toward the Other, this is its essential character." Yet in our efforts to establish intimacy we often seek to eliminate otherness, thereby precluding the space necessary for desire to flourish. We seek intimacy to protect ourselves from feeling alone; and yet creating the distance essential to eroticism means stepping back from the comfort of our partner and feeling more alone.

I suggest that our ability to tolerate our separateness—and the fundamental insecurity it engenders—is a precondition for maintaining interest and desire in a relationship. Instead of always striving for closeness, I argue that couples may be better off cultivating their separate selves. If cultivating separateness sounds harsh, let's think of it instead as nurturing a sense of selfhood. The French psychologist Jacques Salomé talks about the need to develop a personal intimacy with one's own self as a counterbalance to the couple. There is beauty in an image that highlights a connection to oneself, rather than a distance from one's partner. In our mutual intimacy we make love, we have children, and we share physical space and interests. Indeed, we blend the essential parts of our lives. But "essential" does not mean "all." Personal intimacy demarcates a private zone, one that requires tolerance and respect. It is a space—physical, emotional, and intellectual—that belongs only to me. Not everything needs to be revealed. Everyone should cultivate a secret garden.

Love enjoys knowing everything about you; desire needs mystery. Love likes to shrink the distance that exists between me and you, while desire is energized by it. If intimacy grows through repetition and familiarity, eroticism is numbed by repetition. It thrives on the mysterious, the novel, and the unexpected. Love is about having; desire is about wanting. An expression of longing, desire requires ongoing elusiveness. It is less concerned with where it has already been than passionate about where it can still go. But too often, as couples settle into the comforts of love, they cease to fan the flame of desire. They forget that fire needs air.

3

The Pitfalls of Modern Intimacy

Talk Is Not the Only Avenue to Closeness

We have no secrets, we tell each other everything.
—*Carly Simon, "We Have No Secrets"*

WHEN MY MOTHER TALKED ABOUT relationships, she didn't have much to say about intimacy. "You need two things in a marriage," she told me. "You need the will to make it work and you need to be able to make compromises. It's not hard to be right, but then you are right and alone." My father, who was always less pragmatic than my mother, more than filled the quota for expressiveness and demonstrativeness. He openly adored and adorned her with kisses, gifts, and attention. But if I had asked him whether or not they had intimacy, he would have looked at me perplexed, not knowing what I was talking about. He knew love, and he knew partnership, and they implicitly included the vastness of intimacy.

For my parents and others of their generation, the modern discourse on intimacy would have eluded them altogether. Their relationship was far from perfect—they might have come to therapy for any number of reasons—but the notion of "working on their intimacy" would have been alien to them.

When Tevye, in *Fiddler on the Roof*, tells his wife, Golde, that he will allow his daughter to marry the man she loves (instead of the man he has chosen for her), he frames his decision with the understanding that "this is a new world." It's a world where people marry for love, far distant from the world in which he met Golde on their wedding day and was told by his father that he would learn to love her in time. Now, twenty-five years later, as he witnesses the burgeoning love of his daughter, he asks his wife if she does love him, after all these years. Golde answers with an amazing list of experiences they've shared in their life together, and she gives a beautiful and lyrical description of how the "old world" used to think of love and marriage. She washed his clothes, milked his cow, shared his bed, starved with him, fought with him, raised his children, cleaned his house, and cooked his meals. "If that's not love, what is?" she asks. Knowing that Golde loves him doesn't change anything, but Tevye ends the song by acknowledging that "after twenty-five years, it's nice to know."

Golde's picture of marriage doesn't match what we today in the West commonly refer to as intimacy. We'd be more inclined to call it domesticity (at best) or age-old oppression (at worst). In the past, when marriage was a more pragmatic institution, love was optional. Respect was essential. Men and women found emotional connection elsewhere, primarily in same-sex relationships. Men bonded over work and recreation; women connected through child rearing and borrowing sugar. Love within a marriage might develop over time but was not indispensable to the success of the family. Marriage used to be primarily a matter of economic sustenance, and it was a partnership for life. Mating today is a free-choice enterprise, and commitments are built on love. Intimacy has shifted from being a by-product of a long-term relationship to being a mandate for one. In companionate marriage, trust and affection have replaced respect as the relational pillar, bringing us to a place where the centrality of intimacy is unquestioned.

The Ascendance of Intimacy

The family therapist Lyman Wynne points out that "intimacy became recognized as a 'need' only when it became more difficult to achieve." The advent of industrialization and the subsequent rise of urban living touched off a major shift in social structure. Work and family were separated, and so were we: we became more disconnected, more lonely, and more in need of meaningful contact.

In contrast, when people live in close social networks they are more likely to seek space than intimate dialogue. When three generations live under one roof, everyone knows his place; the family members are more apt to abide by rules of formality that ensure privacy and discretion. Though much is shared, everyone gets to stake a claim on something personal—a private corner, a favorite coffee cup, a seat by the window, a quiet read in the loo. From Tokyo to Djibouti to Queens, New York, people who live in an extended family, or who are under the yoke of economic duress and forced to live in close quarters, tend not to seek greater closeness. When people live on top of each other, there is no isolation to transcend, and they are far less interested in embracing western, middle-class ideals of intimacy. Their lives are entwined enough as it is.

Intimacy has become the sovereign antidote for lives of increasing isolation. Our determination to "reach out and touch someone" has reached a peak of religious fervor. Just this morning as I was penning these thoughts my home phone rang; and when I didn't answer, my cell phone chimed in. It was followed immediately by my computer beeping to let me know I had mail. After my private line joined the cacophony, I gave up and allowed myself to be "touched." In our world of instant communication, we supplement our relationships with an assortment of technological devices in the hope that all these gizmos will strengthen our connections. This social frenzy masks a profound hunger for human contact.

Tell Me How You Really Feel

Interestingly, while our need for intimacy has become paramount, the way we conceive of it has narrowed. We no longer plow the land together; today we talk. We have come to glorify verbal communication. I speak; therefore I am. We naively believe that the essence of who we are is most accurately conveyed through words. Many of my own patients wholeheartedly embrace this assumption when they complain, "We're not close. We never talk."

In our era of communication, intimacy has been redefined. No longer is it the deep knowledge and familiarity that develop over time and can be cultivated in silence. Instead, we think of intimacy primarily as a discursive process, one that involves self-disclosure, the trustful sharing of our most personal and private material—our feelings. Of course, it is as much about listening as it is about telling. The receiver of these revelations must be a loving, accepting, nonjudgmental partner—a "good listener," empathetic and validating. We want to feel completely known, deeply recognized, and fully accepted for who we are; and we expect our sharing to be reciprocated.

It is no coincidence that the emergence of modern intimacy, with its emphasis on speech, arose alongside the growing economic independence of women. When women were no longer financially bound to their husbands, nor socially obligated to endure an unhappy union, they began to expect more from marriage. Nonnegotiable drudgery became unacceptable. It was replaced with the expectation of a mutually satisfying emotional connection. The benefits applied to men as well, who were themselves no longer required to be the sole financial providers (it's own form of drudgery).

In our contemporary model of committed coupledom, the female influence is unmistakable. At a time when society needed new narratives of connection, women brought their well-developed communicative resourcefulness. Much ink has been spilled to explain women's superior verbal ability in the emotional arena. For our purposes, suffice it to say that centuries of limited access to power have made us experts in relationship-building. The socialization of girls continues to emphasize the development of relational skills.

More than ever, the lives we lead require tremendous adaptability. We must be able to maintain the connective tissue of our relationships despite the constant pressures of our hectic lives. The feminization of intimacy, with its emphasis on open and honest dialogue, provides the resources necessary to meet the demands of modern relationships.

And the Word Didn't Become Flesh

This having been said, the emphasis on "talk intimacy" is nonetheless problematic, for a number of reasons. The hegemony of the spoken word has veered into a female bias that has, for once, put men in a position of inferiority. Men are socialized to perform, to compete, and to be fearless. The capacity to express feelings is not a prized attribute in the making of American manhood. Dare I say it's not even considered a desirable one?—at least, not yet. When it comes to loving relationships, "talk intimacy" inevitably leaves many men at a loss. In this regime, they suffer from a chronic intimacy deficiency that needs ongoing repair.

So much of masculine identity is predicated on self-control and invulnerability. Yet I have also observed that these very restrictions lead many men to other venues of self-expression. In the absence of a more developed verbal narrative of the self, the body becomes a vital language, a conduit for emotional intimacy. While much has been written about the aggressive manifestations of male sexuality, it is not sufficiently appreciated that the erotic realm also offers men a restorative experience for their more tender side. The body is our original mother tongue, and for a lot of men it remains the only language for closeness that hasn't been spoiled. Through sex, men can recapture the pure pleasure of connection without having to compress their hard-to-articulate needs into the prison of words.

The adherents of talk intimacy (often, though not always, women) have a hard time recognizing these other languages for closeness, hence they feel cheated when their partners are reluctant to confide in them. "Why won't you talk to me?" they plead. "You should be able to tell me anything. Don't you trust me? I want to be your best friend." In this setup, the pressure is always on the non-talker to change, rather than on the talker to be more versatile. This situation minimizes the importance of nonverbal communication: doing nice things for each other, making attentive gestures, or sharing projects in a spirit of collaboration. A priceless smile or a well-timed wink expresses complicity and attunement, especially when words are unavailable.

Eddie, a longtime friend of mine, had a history of getting dumped by women who were dismayed because he couldn't—or wouldn't—"open up." The consensus among these women was that Eddie had a fear of commitment. "Whatever that means," he said. They never knew how he felt about them. He would respond defensively. "What do you mean? I see you every day, don't I? How can you not know how I feel?" When he met his wife, Noriko, she spoke almost no English, and he spoke no Japanese at all. Their courtship was literally speechless. Twelve years later, with two children in tow, he reflects on the early days. "I really think that not being able to talk made this whole thing possible. For once, there was no pressure on me to share. And so Noriko and I had to show how much we liked each other in other ways. We cooked for each other a lot, gave each other baths. I washed her hair. We looked at art. I remember one day I had just seen some amazing sculpture this homeless guy Curtis had made on Lafayette Street—he was crazy but brilliant. Try explaining that in pantomime. Whatever we couldn't say, we showed, so I put her coat on her and led her by the hand all the way across town. Her face lit up when she saw it. It's not like we didn't communicate; we just didn't talk."

When Too Much Is Still Not Enough

I am not convinced that unrestrained disclosure—the ability to speak the truth and not hide anything—necessarily fosters a harmonious and robust intimacy. Any practice can be taken to a ridiculous extreme. Eddie and Noriko remind us that we can be very close without much talk. And the reverse is also true—too much self-revealing talk can still land us on the outskirts of intimacy.

In the wonderful movie *Bliss*, a scene of passionate lovemaking—dim lights, vague body parts, and the roaring groans accompanying orgasm—is immediately followed by a couples therapy session. The therapist, played by Spalding Gray, adheres to an ideology of openness which the husband finds more than a little difficult to take.

Therapist: How's the sex?

Joseph: You go first.

Mary: OK. I have a confession to make. I fake my orgasms. I didn't want to tell you. I didn't want to hurt you.

Joseph: You've never had an orgasm?

Mary:	Not with you.
Therapist:	Joseph, it's important that Mary can tell you how she feels, and for you to be able to hear it.

Obviously, knowing everything about the other, and having him know everything about us, does not always promote the kind of closeness we want. If words serve as venues of connection, they can also stage insuperable obstacles. Needless to say, I don't advocate this kind of therapeutic intervention.

The mandate of intimacy, when taken too far, can resemble coercion. In my own work, I see couples who no longer wait for an invitation into their partner's interiority, but instead demand admittance, as if they are entitled to unrestricted access into the private thoughts of their loved ones. Intimacy becomes intrusion rather than closeness—intimacy with an injunction. "You have to listen to me." "Take care of me; tell me you love me." Something that should develop normally, that is part of the beauty and the wisdom of a loving relationship, is forced on the partner who is less inclined to communicate verbally. In his book *Passionate Marriage*, David Schnarch deftly illustrates how the wish for intimacy can lead a person to impose forced reciprocity as a way to stave off the threat of rejection. The bargain of reciprocity goes something like this: "I'll tell if you will, and I want to, so you have to." We don't like to be intimate alone.

Some couples take this one step farther, confusing intimacy with control. What passes for care is actually covert surveillance—a fact-finding approach to the details of a partner's life. What did you eat for lunch? Who called? What did you guys talk about? This kind of interrogation feigns closeness and confuses insignificant details with a deeper sense of knowledge. I am often amazed at how couples can be up on the minute details of each other's lives, but haven't had a meaningful conversation in years. In fact, such transparency can often spell the end of curiosity. It's as if this stream of questions replaces a more thoughtful and authentically interested inquiry.

When the impulse to share becomes obligatory, when personal boundaries are no longer respected, when only the shared space of togetherness is acknowledged and private space is denied, fusion replaces intimacy and possession co-opts love. It is also the kiss of death for sex. Deprived of enigma, intimacy becomes cruel when it excludes any possibility of discovery. Where there is nothing left to hide, there is nothing left to seek.

Bodies Speak, Too

If one consequence of the supremacy of talk is that it leaves men at a disadvantage, another is that it leaves women trapped in repressed sexuality. It denies the expressive capacity of the female body, and this idea troubles me. Favoring speech as the primary pathway to intimacy reinforces the notion that women's sexual desire is legitimate only when it is embedded in relatedness—only through love can female carnality be redeemed.

Historically, women's sexuality and intellect have never been integrated. Women's bodies were controlled, and their sexuality was contained, in order to avert their corrupting impact on men's virtue. Femininity, associated with purity, sacrifice, and frailty, was a characteristic of the morally successful woman. Her evil twin, the succubus (whore, slut, concubine, witch) was the earthy, sensual, and frankly lusty woman who had traded respectability for sexual exuberance. Vigorous sexuality was the exclusive domain of men. Women have continuously sought to disentangle themselves from the patriarchal split between virtue and lust, and are still fighting this injustice. When we privilege speech and underplay the body, we collude in keeping women confined.

Bilingual Intimacy

When it comes to letting the body speak, Mitch and Laura are at opposite ends of the spectrum. They've reduced their sexual selves to stereotypes. Laura describes Mitch as the classic sex-obsessed man, demanding his rights regardless of how she feels. "The only time he really wants to get close to me is when he wants sex, and he wants it all the time," she says resentfully. Laura, who is strong-willed and sometimes domineering in their everyday interactions, is seen by Mitch as a sexually inhibited woman who repeatedly rejects his advances from some unfathomable feelings of disgust or contempt. "She acts as if I were some sort of crude animal, and shrinks away from me every time I touch her—it makes me feel like shit," he says, sounding bitter.

For Laura, sex is the sum of all the cultural and familial restrictions she absorbed as a child; her body is a gathering place of multiple taboos and anxieties. Like many girls of her generation (she's in her early fifties) she grew up believing that she could be smart or pretty, but not both. The only comments about her looks she remembers from her father were about her developing breasts. And her mother's twisted caution was that she was lucky not to be too pretty, since boys want only one thing. As an adult, she wears concealing clothes—turtlenecks even in the summer—and feels demeaned by compliments about her looks. For her, sexuality evokes fear; she's never been able to enjoy the raptures of her body.

For Mitch, on the other hand, sex is a place where he feels utterly free, uninhibited, and at peace. It wasn't always this way. He was a late bloomer, gawky and not particularly athletic. But he had two things that made his adolescence hopeful: he was a good dancer and he genuinely liked girls. At eighteen he fell in love with Hillary, a college senior with considerable expertise, and his initiation into the voluptuousness of sex was magnificent. Sadly, in his marriage he's come to feel awful about something he'd always experienced with confidence and joy. Meanwhile, Laura has come to feel completely deficient, ungenerous, and guilty.

I encourage Mitch and Laura to listen to each other with greater empathy. Mitch begins to understand that Laura's alienation from her body has nothing to do with him. This eases his sense of rejection and his anguish about being unable to please her. While it is clear to Mitch that his desire is rooted in love, he needs to help Laura trust the sincerity of his interest in her. Far from seeking a selfish discharge, he longs for union.

For her part, Laura learns something equally crucial about Mitch—that when the language of words fails him, as it invariably does in the realm of emotion, he communicates with his body. She'd always felt that Mitch's "itch for the horizontal" had little to do with her; it was just raw physical release. As she hears him, she sees that Mitch needs physicality to voice his tenderness, his yearning to connect. Only in sex does he feel emotionally safe. By limiting him to her own nonphysical language, to the exclusion of his sensual language, Laura has stifled his ability to "speak" to her. She blinds herself to her husband as he really is, and at the same time reinforces the very behaviors she rails against. When Mitch is reduced to using a truncated language of words, the romantic lover disappears and the bully emerges.

Mitch and Laura exemplify two extremes on the mind-body continuum. Couples are often configured on opposite sides of this divide. There are those for whom the body is like a prison in which they feel confined, self-conscious, and self-critical. The body is an inhibited site, awkward and tense. Play and inventiveness have no place there. Words feel safer than gesture and movements, and these people take refuge in speech. When reaching out to others, they prefer the verbal route. Then there are those for whom the body is like a playground, a place where they feel free and unrestricted.

They retain the child's capacity to fully inhabit their bodies. In the physical realm, they can let go; they don't have to be responsible. They are often the partner in the relationship who wants more physical intimacy. It is especially during lovemaking that they are able to escape their inner rumblings. For them, sex is a relief that puts a halt to their anxiety; for their more verbal partners, sex turns out to be a source of anxiety.

As a therapist, I seek to make each partner more fluent in the language of the other. Laura's experience has robbed her of the capacity to recognize the body's vocabulary. Like many women, she battles the age-old repressions of female sexuality that have trapped women in passivity and made us dependent on men to seduce and initiate us into sexuality. Economic and professional independence notwithstanding, Laura remains sexually dependent. She leaves it to Mitch to figure out what she wants. Together, we explore the tortuous conflicts between desire and denial, wanting and not having, gratification and repression. I invite Laura to engage with her fantasies, to own her wanting, and to take responsibility for her sexual fulfillment. I steer her attention to her physical self, and challenge her to break through the vigilance, the guilt, and the disavowal that surround her sexuality. Can she look her mother straight in the eye and still maintain a sense of herself as a sensual being? Can she indulge in her own eroticism and declare the "nice girl" officially void?

When I suggest to Mitch and Laura that they're trapped in a language with too little imagination, an alphabet too limited to contain their erotic life, Mitch bursts into tears. "I'm not angry," he says of all the times that his frustration has led to mean, hurtful words; "I'm heartbroken." I ask Laura to just hold him and I leave the room for a few minutes to give them the chance to connect through the purity of physical touch.

When I return, they're practically falling off opposite ends of the couch, a yawning gulf between them. When I ask what happened, they immediately backslide to the tried and true mutual blame that got them here in the first place. "I tried, but he . . ." "I wouldn't have if she hadn't . . ." I realize that my intervention was more an expression of my own hope than any intention on their part. They weren't ready.

Realizing the futility of any more talk, in the months that followed I tried several different approaches, most of which relied on physical interactions rather than verbal ones. I had them lead each other around the room, trying out different arrangements of leaders and followers: cooperation, resistance, and passivity. I had them fall backward into each other's waiting arms. I had them stand face-to-face and push against each other with their open hands. I had them mirror each other's movements. The conversations that followed the games became gradually more revealing, less critical, and even more playful. By giving a physical but nonsexual representation to their emotional impasse, they were able to see their patterns of resistance.

"I can let him get close," Laura admits, "but not too close. I trust him, but only so much. I always hold back, don't I?"

"When you doubt your own desirability, it is harder to trust Mitch's desire for you." I explain. "It's far easier to locate the fault with him—and, to be fair, he gives you plenty to work with—than it is to face the depth of your own self-doubt."

Mitch, who had been pointing to Laura's sexual passivity for years, had some realizations of his own. "I guess I'm not too creative, either. When we were doing the exercise, I felt uncomfortable taking the lead. I hate to admit it, but I liked the passive resistance most. I'm unbeatable at that one." I reminded Mitch that when he met Hillary, his first love, she too took the lead. "You do indeed express yourself with great eloquence in the physical realm, but you're highly dependent on a powerful interlocutor to make it safe for you. So far, Laura hasn't been that."

When Mitch and Laura came to me, I was reluctant to take

them on. They considered me the therapist of last resort; I was either the third or the fifth (I can't remember which) they had consulted in more than two decades. For years, they had been trying to talk their way out of their rut. Evidently, it hadn't worked. Instead they were engaged in a verbal thrust-and-parry, defensive, hostile, and totally fused. They had had plenty of self-disclosure, but it was far from intimate.

I knew enough not to limit myself to the habits of the talking cure—talking had become squawking and was going nowhere. The exercises provided an alternative lens to examine their dynamics. The physicalization of their problems gave us a fresh text to read together. It was novel enough to jar them, and to interrupt their entrenchment. They were stretching into new territory.

In my work with patients I stress that intimacy isn't monolithic; nor is it always consistent. It is intermittent, meant to wax and wane even in the best relationships. The family therapist Kaethe Weingarten steers us away from looking at intimacy as a static feature of a relationship; she sees it instead as a quality of interaction that takes place in isolated moments and that exists both within and without long-term commitment. There's the synchronization of dance partners, the sudden identification between strangers on a plane, the solidarity of witnesses to a catastrophe, the mutual recognition of survivors—of breast cancer, alcoholism, terrorism, divorce. There's the intimacy between professionals and those they serve—doctor and patient, therapist and client, stripper and regular. While we expect to experience these discrete moments of recognition in ongoing relationships, they are not necessarily bound to any overarching narrative. They can be circumstantial, spontaneous, and without follow-up. Informed by Weingarten's ideas, I no longer look at relationships as being either intimate or not. Instead, I track each couple's ability to engage in a series of intimate bids tendered over time.

Sometimes the emotional weaving is done through talk; often, it is not. Building a bookshelf for your lover, changing the snow tires on your wife's car, and learning to make his mom's chicken soup all carry the promise of connection. Golde in *Fiddler on the Roof* reminds us that even ordinary daily activities will, over time, weave themselves into a rich tapestry of connection. Eddie and Noriko, masters of nonverbal communication, can teach us all a lesson in alternative ways to express our love. When we value only what is disclosed through words, we do ourselves a disservice. At a time when we could use just about any way to connect, we need to honor and recognize the many ways we can reach out and touch someone.

4

Democracy Versus Hot Sex
Desire and Egalitarianism Don't Play by the Same Rules

No bill of sexual rights can hold its own against the lawless, untamable landscape of the erotic imagination.
—*Daphne Merkin*

SEVERAL YEARS AGO I ATTENDED a presentation at a national conference where the speaker discussed a couple who had come to therapy in part because of a sharp decline in their sexual activity. Previously, they had acted out fantasies of domination and submission; now, following the birth of their second child, the wife wanted more conventional sex. But the husband was attached to their old style of lovemaking, so they were stuck. The presenter took the approach that resolving this couple's sexual difficulty was going to require working through the emotional dynamics of their marriage and their new status as parents. But in the discussion that followed, the audience proved far less interested in the couple's overall relationship than in the disconcerting presence of domination and submission in their erotic life.

What pathology, several participants asked, might underlie the man's need to sexually objectify his wife, and her desire for bondage in the first place? Perhaps, some people speculated, motherhood had restored her sense of dignity, so that now she refused to be so demeaned. Some suggested that the impasse reflected long-standing gender differences: men tend to pursue separateness, power, and control, while women yearn for loving affiliation and connection. Still others were certain that couples like this needed more empathetic connection to counteract their tendency to engage in an implicitly abusive, power-driven relationship. What these remarks made clear was the unspoken subtext that such practices are inherently degrading to women, a rebuke to the very idea of gender equality, and antithetical to a good, healthy marriage.

After two hours of talking about sex, the group had not once mentioned pleasure or eroticism, so I finally spoke up. I wondered, I said, if I was the only one surprised by this omission. After all, the sex had been entirely consensual. Maybe the woman no longer wanted to be tied up by her husband because now she had a baby continually attached to her breasts, binding her more effectively than ropes ever could. Didn't people in the audience have their own sexual preferences, preferences they didn't feel the need to interpret or justify? Why automatically assume that there had to be something degrading and pathological about this couple's erotic play? More to the point, I wondered, was a woman's ready participation in submission too great a challenge for the politically correct? Was it too threatening to conceive of a strong, secure woman enjoying acting out sexual fantasies of submission? Would such recognition lessen women's moral authority? Perhaps the participants in this conference were afraid that if women did reveal such desires, they'd somehow sanction male dominance everywhere—in business, professional life, politics, and economics. Maybe the very ideas of sexual dominance and submission, conquest and subjugation, aggression and surrender (regardless of which partner plays which part) can't be squared with the ideals of fairness, compromise, and equality that undergird marriage today.

As a relative outsider with regard to American society, I suspected that the attitudes I saw in this meeting reflected deeper cultural assumptions. Did the clinicians in the room believe that this couple's sexual practices, even though consensual and completely nonviolent, were too wild and "kinky," and therefore inappropriate and irresponsible for the ponderously serious business of maintaining a marriage and raising a family? It was as if sexual pleasure and eroticism that strayed onto slightly outré paths of fantasy and play, particularly games involving aggression and power, must be stricken from the repertoire of responsible adults in loving, committed relationships.

After the conference, I engaged in many intense conversations with couples therapists from South America, the Middle East, and Europe. We realized that we all felt somewhat out of step with American sexual attitudes, but putting a finger on what was culturally different wasn't easy. On a subject as laden with taboos as the expression of sexuality, making generalizations is a slippery slope. But if I could hazard one unpolished observation, I would say that egalitarianism, directness, and pragmatism are entrenched in American culture and inevitably influence the way we think about and experience love and sex. Latin Americans' and Europeans' attitudes toward love, on the other hand, tend to reflect other cultural values, and are more likely to embody the dynamics of seduction, the focus on sensuality, and the idea of complementarity (i.e., being different but equal) rather than absolute sameness.

Bedroom Politics

Some of America's best features—the belief in democracy, equality, consensus-building, compromise, fairness, and mutual tolerance—can, when carried too punctiliously into the bedroom, result in very boring sex. Sexual desire and good citizenship don't play by the same rules. And while enlightened egalitarianism represents one of the greatest advances of modern society, it can exact a toll in the erotic realm.

Elizabeth spent twenty years shepherding Vito from the machismo traditions of southern Italy to the postfeminist equality of suburban New York. When he says, "I think we're partnering better," in a voice that still sounds like Don Vito Corleone's, I know just how much cultural transformation has taken place. Elizabeth is a woman in her mid-forties who describes herself as "hyperresponsible." She's a school psychologist who oversees the well-being of more than 400 elementary school children in addition to being in charge of most things in her own home. "I've always done the right thing. I've always been very task-oriented. I'll make a list and keep it. In some ways it's always worked. And I've always been in relationships where being the coordinator, competent and in control, was my designated job. There didn't seem to be any time when I could just let myself go, feel free and giddy and maybe even a little irresponsible" Elizabeth pauses and smiles shyly. "Then I met Vito and discovered just how much I'm drawn to sexual submission. It may not fit the way I always thought of myself, or the way others thought of me, but it's the truth."

"Because sex is a place where you can safely lose control?" I ask.

"Yes."

"It is the one area where you don't have to make any decisions, where you don't have to feel responsible for anyone else."

"For me it's like a vacation," she explains. "I don't have to wear makeup; I don't have to answer the phone; I don't have to be in charge. It's like being on a wonderful, distant island, far away from my ordinary life. I can just step out of my world and be somebody else, sexy and a little wild." Elizabeth wants to be manhandled, told what to do—as if, through her erotic self, she can correct an imbalance in her life and replenish something vital. She delights in the abandon that comes with the sense of powerlessness. And I would add that she also gets a charge from playing in the forbidden zone of inequality.

"When he comes on to me forcefully, it makes me feel sexy. It heightens the tension. Like he wants me so much he just can't help himself," Elizabeth says. Vito, quick to respond, adds, "She can't help herself, either. When she gives in, I know I'm irresistible."

The harsh realities of violence, rape, sexual trafficking, child pornography, and hate crimes require that we keep a tight rein on the abuses of power that pervade the politics of sex. The poetics of sex, however, are often politically incorrect, thriving on power plays, role reversals, unfair advantages, imperious demands, seductive manipulations, and subtle cruelties. American men and women, shaped by the feminist movement and its egalitarian ideals, often find themselves challenged by these contradictions. We fear that playing with power imbalances in the sexual arena, even in a consensual relationship between mature adults, risks overthrowing the respect that is essential to human relationships.

By no means am I calling for a reversal of history or an anti-feminist agenda. Any discussion of modern-day couples and sexuality would be perversely wrongheaded if it did not recognize the enormous and vastly salutary influence of feminism on the shape of American family life. The women's movement sought to eliminate deep-rooted gender inequalities and to unearth the structures that perpetuated male domination in all spheres of life, including sexuality. It challenged the double standard that encouraged sexual experimentation by men, even seeing it as a necessary developmental stage, but forbade that same curiosity in women. This same double standard demanded sexual loyalty from women, while turning a blind eye on roaming men because "That's how men are." (There are still countries today where a man can murder his unfaithful wife with no legal repercussions whatsoever. In some cultures, killing her is the only way to restore his honor and that of his family.)

Gender differences and their ensuing taboos and prohibitions had long been viewed as categorical imperatives, biologically rooted and therefore immutable. Feminism showed that these undisputed truisms and characterizations were, in fact, social constructions that reinforced a long-standing gender ordering—one that obviously favored men. Books like *Our Bodies, Ourselves* and *The Women's Room* aimed to restore a sense of sexual ownership to women, both legally and psychologically, and to free them from the constraints that had governed female sexuality. Female sexual pleasure could not be set free until women were relatively safe from the traditional and very real dangers associated with sex. Sexually transmitted diseases, rape, and unwanted pregnancy brought not only shame but also ruination, and childbirth always carried the threat of fatality.

Early feminists were much more interested in the subject of sexual sovereignty than in the subject of pleasure. First things first, they thought. As long as men completely dominate business and political life, as long as women are economically dependent on men, as long as the burden of child care falls wholly on women's shoulders (toppling even the most egalitarian couples), you cannot speak of a liberated female sexuality. Undeniably, American feminists achieved momentous improvements in all these aspects of women's lives; and no real freedom, sexual or other, is conceivable without them.

But these improvements also smuggled in some unintended consequences. Without denigrating those historically significant achievements, I do believe that the emphasis on egalitarian and respectful sex—purged of any expressions of power, aggression, and transgression—is antithetical to erotic desire for men and women alike.

The Bounded Space of Eroticism

Elizabeth and Vito have worked hard to have an equitable marriage, but sex takes them to another place. The power differential that would be unacceptable in her emotional relationship with Vito is precisely what excites Elizabeth erotically. At first, when she discloses her sexual predilection, she is embarrassed. It doesn't fit her image of herself as a liberated, powerful woman. "I've struggled to accept what turns me on. For a long time I was disturbed by my fantasies. Submission just isn't me. It took me years to reconcile what arouses me with my political beliefs. Somewhere in the midst of marriage, kids, and career, I realized that it was time to stop hiding, to stop pretending, and most of all to stop apologizing for who I was and what I hungered for in the world. Getting older helps. I don't feel as if I have to justify myself. Maybe that's the meaning of sexual liberation."

A lot of women find their desire for sexual submission hard to accept. But stepping out of ourselves is exactly what eroticism allows us to do. In eros, we trample on cultural restrictions; the prohibitions we so vigorously uphold in the light are often the ones we enjoy transgressing in the dark. It's an alternative space where we can safely experience our taboos. The erotic imagination has the force to override reason, convention, and social barriers.

The more I point to the tensions in these epiphanies of pleasure, the more relieved Elizabeth seems. I continue, "Of course nothing is scarier than a true loss of control in 'reality.' But the point of fantasy is that it allows you to transcend the moral and psychological constraints of your everyday life." In the liberating expression of sexuality we give in to our unruly impulses and the disavowed, lurid parts of ourselves. Mordechai Gafni, a scholar of Jewish mysticism, explains that fantasies are like mirrors. We hold them in front of us in order to see what is behind. We spot images of ourselves that are otherwise inaccessible. If commitment requires a trade-off of freedom for security, then eroticism is the gateway back to freedom. In the broad expansiveness of our imagination we uncover the freedom that allows us to tolerate the confines of reality.

The very dynamics of power and control that can be challenging in an emotional relationship can, when eroticized, become highly desirable. In the crucible of the erotic mind, we bring the more vexing components of love—dependency, surrender, jealousy, aggression, even hostility—and transform them into powerful sources of excitement. My patient Oscar can't stand being told what to do by his bossy wife, yet he enjoys being tossed around by her sexually. When she barks orders about the dishes, the experience takes him back to his mom's kitchen. But he does not feel this regressive threat once the lights have been turned off. What he loathes in the domestic sphere becomes his choice in the erotic. Maxwell, who keeps a shrewd eye on his beautiful girlfriend's many admirers, repeatedly brings them up when he makes love to her. What threatens in public becomes enchantment in private. He parlays his daily fears into nightly seductions. And Elizabeth, the take-charge woman, loves to get a break when Vito takes over sexually. She does not experience his control as oppressive. On the contrary, she feels taken care of. And she feels a renewed respect for him when, "For a change, he knows what to do." His control offers her a safe container in which she can release her lusty self. The imbalance of power is both safe and sexy—at once protective and liberating.

Subverting Power

Some would say that Elizabeth's desire for submission is nothing more than a reenactment of traditional male domination. They would claim that sexual arrangements in which one partner is dominant and controlling, the other passive and weak, are inherently hierarchical and oppressive, nothing more than a sexist replay of patriarchy. But prisoners rarely have the desire to pretend they are prisoners. Only the free can choose to make believe. To my thinking, being able to play with roles goes some way toward indicating that you're no longer controlled by them. Play has the potential to disrupt the very notion of gender categorization. For Elizabeth, being controlled sexually is itself a subversive act that is ultimately liberating. The same is true for Marcus, who heads the research and development unit of a large international software company. He is a classic type A man: competitive, ambitious, spending more time in the air than on the ground. His tough-mindedness and aggressiveness have made him a natural leader in his highly competitive field. The word "power" is attached to many of his activities and often turns up in his conversation. He takes power walks, drinks power drinks, does power lunches, and recharges during ten-minute power naps. And in his free time, he likes a good spanking.

When Marcus arrives at the house of his girlfriend, it's after a long day of being the boss. With a sexually powerful woman, a dominating woman, he gets a respite from having to be in control. With his girlfriend in charge, in the role of dominatrix, he can give it up, for he knows that she can withstand the intensity of his urges. The surrender not only pleases him erotically, it nurtures him emotionally as well. Like Elizabeth, Marcus gets to experience a submerged but vital facet of himself in the erotic mirror. In our culture, passivity is perceived as female and weak. Consequently, it generates great emotional conflict for men (and for many women). But that doesn't eradicate it from our psyche, or make it any less desirable. Marcus fears surrender as much as he craves it. His fantasy permits a bounded passivity, a safe but masked return to the mother's arms. And while he is not interested in intellectual or heavy-duty psychological explanations of his "motivation," his erotic inclinations challenge the stereotypical power distribution that always sees the man on top.

There Is No Love Without Hate

The defenders of modern intimacy—with marital counselors and self-help authors on the front line—have continuously sought to neutralize the thorny issue of power in committed relationships. The ideal partnership is said to be one of absolute equality in every area of the relationship, as if, with scale in hand, we could measure power quantitatively. Many of us, steeped in this ideology of fairness and mutuality, want nothing less.

But the fact is that negotiating power is part and parcel of all human relationships. We recognize it most easily when it's expressed outright, through authority, coercion, bullying, aggression, and castigation. The powerful one metes out punishments and rewards depending on one's degree of compliance with his or her wishes. But there is also the power of the weak. Deference, passivity, withholding, ingratiation, and the moral one-upmanship of the victim are their own manifestations of might. Power and power imbalances are inescapable.

Ethel Spector Person, in *Feeling Strong*, writes that we first learn about power differentials in the power grid of our families. "All power relationships, all desires either to dominate or submit, have their psychological roots in the fact that we were all once little children with big parents, and their existential roots in our feelings of being small people in an out-of-control big world that we need to be able to tame." Childhood is our basic training for power tactics. We have our will; our parents have theirs. We demand; they object. We bargain for what we want; they tell us what we can have. We learn to resist, and we learn to surrender. At best we learn to balance, to mediate, to understand.

All these permutations of power stumble into our adult intimacies, and gender does matter. Boys and girls undergo a radically different initiation in wielding power. Men become adept at direct expressions of power, women at indirect expressions; and these differences are discernible in our sexual scripts.

As adults, we seek control in part as a defense against the vulnerability inherent in love. When we put our hopes on one person, our dependence soars. So do our frustrations and disappointments. The greater our helplessness, the more dangerous the threat of humiliation. The more we need, the angrier we are when we don't get. Kids know this; lovers do, too. No one can bring us to the boiling point as quickly as our partner (except maybe our parents, the original locus of dependent rage). Love is always accompanied by hate.

While we fear the depth of our dependence, many of us are even more frightened by the depth of our rage. We resort to intricate relational contortions in order to keep all this combustion in check. Yet the couples who most successfully implement this model of placidity are rarely passionate lovers. When we confuse assertion with aggression, neutralize otherness, adjust our longings, and reason away our hostility, we assemble a calmness that is reassuring but not very exciting. Stephen Mitchell makes the point that the capacity to contain aggression is a precondition for the capacity to love. We must integrate our aggression rather than eradicate it. He explains, "The degradation of romance, the waning of desire, is due not to the contamination of love by aggression, but to the inability to sustain the necessary tension between them."

Jed and Coral

Jed is unassuming. He is a clean-shaven, mild-mannered architect, brilliant and well-spoken. He is kind, never the sort of person to get in your face about anything. But sexually, he's another man. Jed discovered S-M (sadomasochism) as a teenager, and for years he has used eroticism as a venue for aggression. He loves leather, hard surfaces, chains, handcuffs. "I used to be shy, and it was hard for me to assert myself. But at the same time I was angry a lot, and I didn't know where to go with it. I was too afraid of hurting people, so I kept it all inside."

"I can see why S-M was so attractive to you," I reply. "You could make demands and not fear hurting anyone. The unambiguous codes, the negotiating beforehand, made it safe for you. Emotionally, you tend to put other people first. Sexual domination is a way for you to override the other person's supremacy. It's a clever answer to your more typical emotional subordination."

"Exactly," he says. "But at the same time, you know, it's all about their needs. I'm pleasing them—that's the key piece. They want it. They have to be really into it, or it's a no-go for me."

For years, Jed avoided getting serious with women. Becoming close felt obliterating. Haunted by the timid little boy he once was, he dreaded feeling powerless and dependent. "Coral was the first woman I ever loved who I didn't feel indebted to. I wasn't constantly on guard not to be sucked up by the relationship."

Jed grew up as a loner, had few friends, and spent much of his adolescence reading science fiction and listening to heavy metal in his room. Coral, who grew up in the same neighborhood, barely remembers him from high school. She was popular, pretty, outgoing. She edited the yearbook. "I wasn't on the A-list, but I had a perfectly respectable place." Even today, Coral has many friends. She is the hub of her social circle, and she has plenty of interests to supplement her rising career as a documentary filmmaker.

Eleven years after graduating from high school they ran into each other at a wedding. Jed had learned to mask his shyness with satire, and Coral was drawn to his perceptiveness and offbeat sense of humor. Not to be dismissed was the fact that he had turned into a really handsome guy. She made sure to leave the party with his phone number, for she knew it would be up to her to make the first move. They started dating, and they have been together for six years.

Jed and Coral are wonderfully compatible in most areas of their life, but sexually they have very different sensibilities. "I don't understand where his motives come from," she says. "I've never come across this before, and I've been with plenty of men, and there are plenty of kinky things that excite me. I just don't get this—maybe because I grew up in this very feminist world of political correctness and respect for women. In a way I feel disrespected. It feels cheap, tawdry, and it makes me feel like . . ."

"Like a slut?" I ask her.

"No, I don't think there's anything wrong with being a slut. I was a slut for a long time. It just makes me feel less desirable. I don't feel like it's about me. It doesn't have anything to do with me and therefore I don't feel connected with it or motivated by it or interested in it. Does that makes sense?"

"Yeah, it makes sense," Jed answers, "but for me, I don't see it as forgetting you, forgetting your identity. For me, I see it as I'm honoring you by being willing to completely step outside my armor of defense and say, 'Well, I trust you enough to show you this.'"

In order for us to move forward, Jed and Coral each need a stronger sense of where the other is coming from. We do an exercise in which they divide a piece of paper by drawing a line down the middle, then separately write their immediate associations of the word "love" on the left-hand side. I give them prompts: "When I think of love, I think of . . ." "When I love I feel . . ." "When I am loved I feel . . ." "In love, I look for . . ." As soon as they finish, they write their answers to the next set of prompts on the right-hand side: "When I think of sex I think . . ." "When I desire, I feel . . ." "When I am desired, I feel . . ." "In sex, I look for . . ."

This exercise, though simple, is remarkably illuminating. First, because it lays out exactly how love and desire are parsed in each partner's mind—how separate they are and how interwoven. Second, it enables me to look at the congruence of these arrangements between partners. As I suspected, Jed and Coral experience sex in opposing ways, and they look to sex for different things. Coral seeks intimate connection through sex, and love charges her desire. She associates love with warmth and security. Being loved makes her feel safe. Being wanted does the same. For her, sex is sanguine, wholesome, luxe. "I've connected with every person I've had sex with. Even in one-night stands I would walk away smiling, thinking I was in love. I had to learn that sex and love aren't always the same thing, that I didn't have to want to marry every man I slept with."

For Jed, intimate connection emerges after the fact, and love and sex don't blend nearly as seamlessly as they do for Coral. Love feels safe, but also confining. It is laced with conflict. "I feel like I have to restrict what I do and say to avoid hurting her. I feel vulnerable, exposed, and disoriented. It's painful. I think I may not deserve it because I just don't feel worth it. It's still hard to see sometimes what inspires her to love me. I'm anxious." But when it comes to sex, he has an entirely different experience. "Sex has always fascinated me. It's the one place I can really be myself, where I can express all kinds of feelings I usually keep under wraps. Sex is deeply entwined with power; they're not fully distinct for me." Aggression is an intrinsic part of his sexuality. It emboldens him. He doesn't need to subordinate himself to the woman's needs or feelings; nor does he get lost in them. "I need the power because I felt so powerless for so long in my life. I need to compartmentalize."

"When the emotional connection is too intense it hinders the sex because you start confining yourself. The same confining you described in the 'love' column." I suggest.

"If I care about her too much, I can't risk exposing my aggression. I care about what she thinks of me, see? The person can't be too close to me, or I feel threatened. I need distance to be turned on."

Jed is trying to map out the structure of his sexuality for

Coral. Aggression is the initial motivator, but the real sexual charge is the autonomy that aggression permits him. "It's about how manners don't matter anymore. What other people think doesn't matter anymore. Dignity doesn't matter anymore. All there is is need, animal desire. It's freedom, which I've been fighting for my whole life."

Let's face it: Jed and Coral aren't an ideal sexual fit. And it's possible that this part of their relationship will never become *Nine and 1/2 Weeks*. Yet each time they've considered parting, they've realized that they may find a better sexual match, but not a better life partner.

Here's the direction I took. Given Jed's ability to feel mastery largely in sexual dominance, I endorsed Coral's request that she experience some of Jed's assertiveness beyond the bedroom. "Part of what makes this so weird for me is that Jed is incredibly passive in every other aspect of our life. The contrast is totally jarring. I wish he were more decisive and less deferential generally." I encourage Jed to start making some claims outside the sexual arena. He's a novice at this kind of assertiveness. Choosing a restaurant or a movie is hard for him; telling her he wants to stay in New York for Thanksgiving (and not see her entire extended family, as they do every year) is almost impossible. I never suggest to Jed that he needs to reconfigure his sexuality. But I do urge him to learn to wield power in other areas of his life as well. It's important for Jed to know that his wants will be honored outside the rituals of S-M.

By the same token, he wouldn't mind it if Coral transferred some of her directorial boldness from the editing room to their four-poster bed. Jed makes the point that Coral, too, could bring some assertiveness to their sex life. "When you finish brushing your teeth and putting on your pajamas, and then you ask me if we're going to have sex tonight in this matter-of-fact, nudging way, it just doesn't do anything for me. I need more of a charge. Tell me you want me, unzip my pants, walk naked into the room. Something, anything, besides, 'Are we going to have sex tonight?' I do it for you. I light the candles, create the mood you like, make love to you slowly. I do the vanilla for you. I try; you don't."

For Coral's part, she may never like Jed's sexual kinks, but I encourage her to be open to understanding them. By holding court, judging him, and failing to grasp his red-light tastes, she's condemned to feeling demeaned. Sadly, she fails to see that Jed is actually taking a big risk by trusting her to enter the primal bog of his erotic self.

Rebalancing the "Dominant" Culture

Most fans of kinky sex, at least those I've encountered, are drawn by the erotics of power and not, as it may appear to an outsider, by violence or pain. In fact, the carefully negotiated contracts, which specify what can and cannot be done, by whom, to whom, and for how long, are meant to guarantee both pleasure and safety. You submit only as much as you're willing; you dominate only as far as you're allowed.

In the parallel universe of sex, power bids become a plaything, an experiment, a way to temporarily experience relations we're loath to inhabit in real life. If, in our daily life, we shun dependence, in our erotic life we might welcome it. If it is our aggression that makes us twitch with discomfort, sexual enactments can permit a safe experience of power. Whether our real-life aversion is to submission, as it is for Elizabeth, or to autonomy, as it is for Jed, the sexual drama can offer catharsis.

For years S-M and D-S (domination and submission) were fringe behaviors that roamed on the outskirts of conventional sexuality. They were primarily a practice of gay men, who tended to be more successful than heterosexuals at isolating sexual aggression for the purpose of pleasure (as the sociologist Anthony Giddens notes). In recent years these marginal practices have moved into the mainstream. A growing number of citizens in the early twenty-first century—gay and straight, male and female, left and right, urban and suburban—get their sexual kicks from giving and taking orders. There are far too many of them to fit a minority psychological profile.

The social critic Camille Paglia sees this rise in domination and submission as a collective fantasy that tweaks the rough spots of our egalitarian culture. It seems to me that rituals of domination and submission are a subversive way to put one over on a society that glorifies control, belittles dependency, and demands equality. In cultures where these values are at a premium—America, for example—we find more and more people seeking to give up control, revel in dependency, and recognize the very inequities no one wants to talk about. Seen in this light, sex clubs are havens of acceptance for what society rejects. This explicit exchange of power, which transfers freely and consensually from one party to another, is a far cry from the rigid distribution of power that pervades our society. In real life, power is much harder to negotiate, and almost impossible either to acquire or to relinquish. No one wants to give up her piece of the pie.

I am keenly aware of the disparities of power that pervade our society, and not a day goes by when I am not witness to the real fallout of intimate violence. But I also know that aggression, as a human emotion, cannot be purged from human interactions, especially not among those who love each other. Aggression is the shadow side of love. It is also an intrinsic component of sexuality, and it can never be entirely excised from sexual relationships.

In my work with couples, I aim to uncover dynamics of power. I try to make them manifest, to examine the tensions, and to redress the inequities. I also look at the harmonious imbalances unique to each couple. Not all inequities are a source of trouble. Sometimes these form a couple's basis of harmony. I don't seek just to neutralize power; I also seek to harness it. Together, we look for ways to express it safely, creatively, fearlessly, and sexually.

5

Can Do!

The Protestant Work Ethic Takes On the Degradation of Desire

Energy and persistence conquer all things.

—Benjamin Franklin

IN MATTERS OF LOVE, AS in much else, America is a goal-oriented society. We prefer explicit meanings, candor, and plain speech to imponderables, ambiguity, and allusion. We rely on the concreteness of words to convey our feelings and needs, rather than on more subtle avenues to closeness. "Get to the point." "Spit it out." "Don't beat around the bush." America invented assertiveness training. This penchant for clarity and unvarnished directness is encouraged by many therapists as well: "If you want to make love to your partner, why don't you say it clearly? And tell him or her exactly what you want."

We believe that with a well-defined goal, a good plan, solid organizational skills, and hard work, anything is possible. This is the idea behind Americans' optimism. With the right effort and unbending determination, there is no obstacle you can't overcome. Hard work is rewarded by success. Conversely, if you fail, you probably are lazy, unmotivated, self-indulgent, and unwilling to really try to get what you want. You lack "spunk," and you have only yourself to blame. And there's no reason why this booster-ish, essentially entrepreneurial interpretation wouldn't extend to any existential or romantic quandary as well. Apply this business model to romance, and you get books like *Find a Husband After 35 Using What I Learned at Harvard Business School*, by Rachel Greenwald; *5 Minutes to Orgasm Every Time You Make Love*, by Claire D. Hutchins; and *Seven Weeks to Better Sex*, by Domeena Renshaw. Americans cherish the capacity to define what we desire and then score: if you know what you want in your relationship, just go for it. Nailing it down to an exact number of steps, not exceeding ten, promises you entrance into the garden of earthly delights with hardly a minute wasted.

As a European, I have always admired Americans' optimism. It is the opposite of the fatalism and resignation that pervade so many other, more traditional cultures, and it expresses a healthy sense of entitlement. People here don't like to say, "That's just the way it is; you can't change it."

But this can-do attitude encourages us to assume that dwindling desire is an operational problem that can be fixed. From magazine articles to self-help books, we are encouraged to view a lack of sex in our relationships as a scheduling issue that demands better pri-oritizing and time management, or as a consequence of poor com-munication. If the problem is testosterone deficiency, we can get a prescription—an excellent technical solution. For the sexual mal-aise that can't be so easily medicalized, remedies abound: books, videos, and sexual accoutrements are there to assist you not only with the basics, but to bring you to unimagined levels of ecstasy. In her book *Against Love*, Laura Kipnis writes:

> *Whole new sectors of the economy have been spawned,*
> *an array of ancillary industries and markets fostered, and*
> *massive social investments in new technologies undertaken,*

from Viagra to couples porn: late-capitalism's Lourdes for dying marriages. Like dedicated doctors keeping corpses breathing with shiny heart-lung machines and artificial organs, couples too, armed with their newfangled technologies, can now beat back passion's death.

This pragmatic approach typifies how the great country of manifest destiny goes about solving problems. You break the problem down to its component parts, study each one, and come up with a step-by-step plan that you can work on, a solution that promises calculable results. Apply this to sexual problems, though, and you get a model that focuses more on sexual functioning than on sexual feeling. The sex therapist Leonore Tiefer cautions us that in this paradigm, the body is divvied into a collection of unrelated parts, and satisfaction is seen as a result of their perfect functioning.

This emphasis on physical achievement rather than desire and pleasure goes hand in hand with an emphasis on genitals, and reinforces the dominant male orientation. The penis is the new patient, having replaced its human owner, and the ability to achieve and maintain a steely erection overshadows any other kind of sexual proficiency. With Viagra, sex is too easily reduced to erections. (And the search is on for a female Viagra—good news for all the helpful husbands currently trading housework for sex, but bad news for the wives who see their own lack of desire as having more to do with romance than with tumescence.) The subjective experience of sexual pleasure is replaced by an objective list of criteria that is easily indexed but woefully truncated: erection, intercourse, orgasm.

Sexuality is besieged by quantification that provides statistics against which we can compare our own relationships to see if we measure up. *Newsweek* magazine tells us that the experts currently define a sexless marriage as one in which couples have sex no more than ten times a year. Those who have sex eleven times in a twelve-month period can breathe a sigh of relief. The rest must count themselves among the 15 to 20 percent of normative sexless couples. We've become exceedingly preoccupied with frequency of sexual activity and number of orgasms. How much sex? How intense is the sex? What's the level of performance? The more diffuse and uncrunchable aspects of sexual expression—love, intimacy, power, surrender, sensuality, and excitement—rarely make it to the front page of a newspaper or the cover of a magazine. Eroticism as an immeasurable quality of aliveness and imagination is reduced to what the French author Jean-Claude Guillebaud calls *une arithmétique physiologique*—a physiological arithmetic.

But when we reduce sex to a function, we also invoke the idea of dysfunction. We are no longer talking about the art of sex; rather, we are talking about the mechanics of sex. Science has replaced religion as the authority; and science is a more formidable arbiter. Medicine knows how to scare even those who scoff at religion. Compared with a diagnosis, what's a mere sin? We used to moralize; today we normalize, and performance anxiety is the secular version of our old religious guilt.

In my experience, a treatment that places a premium on performance and reliability often exacerbates the very problems it purports to solve. The "sexual performance perfection industry" generates its own inhibitions and anxieties. More often than not, the beauty and flow of a sexual encounter unfurl in a safe, noncompetitive, and non-result-oriented atmosphere. Sensuality simply doesn't lend itself to the rigors of scorekeeping.

This is not to say that practical advice and expert solutions are never useful or necessary. If you have poor communication, of course you should work at it; if you're too busy for sex, you're too busy. If you lack knowledge, inform yourself. If you have a problematic physical condition—age, hormonal changes, diabetes, prostate cancer, hysterectomy—find a doctor who can offer medical support. There are many books that offer sound help in this area. But while the problem-solving model addresses important aspects of our sexual contretemps, it fails to take on the quixotic and fundamentally existential issues of human eroticism that are far beyond any neat technical fix.

When Work Doesn't Work

We are indeed a nation that prides itself on efficiency. But here's the catch: eroticism is inefficient. It loves to squander time and resources. As Adam Phillips wryly notes, "In our erotic life work does not work . . . trying is always trying too hard. Eroticism is an imaginative act, and you can't measure it. We glorify efficiency and fail to recognize that the erotic space is a radiant interlude in which we luxuriate, indifferent to demands of productivity; pleasure is the only goal. Octavio Paz writes, "The moment of merging is a crack in time, a balm against the wounds inflicted by the minutes and hours of time. A moment totally eternal as it is ephemeral." It is a leap into a world beyond.

This leap entails a loss of control that we're taught from a very young age to guard against. We are socialized to tame our primal side: our unruly impulses, our sexual urges, and our rapacious appetites. Social order is built on this restraint, and lack thereof threatens to create chaos. Because loss of control is almost exclusively seen in a negative light, we don't even entertain the idea that surrender can be emotionally or spiritually enlightening. But experiencing a temporary suspension of our discernible self is often liberating and expansive. I have seen many people stumble when they can't simply take the problem of eros and fix it. They are left feeling bewildered and frightened by their slackened command. I help them learn how to relinquish control intentionally, as a means of personal growth and self-discovery.

Ryan and Christine have been in therapy for a year. I meet with them together and individually as they struggle through the transition from being a sexually entwined couple to being the parents of three small children. Following the birth of their twin daughters, the lovers' erotic inspiration began gasping for air. While some couples accept fading intensity with gracious resignation, settling into affectionate companionship, Ryan and Christine don't want to give up. The memory of what they once had is still dear to them. They make a clear distinction between having sex and making love, and they haven't made love in a while. They've rented videos, they've taken baths together, and they are committed to their weekly date. They've tried a lot of things, some yielding satisfying results, others a total waste. Merely having sex is not really their issue. Of course they'd like to have it more often, but their concern is more about intensity than frequency. It's not the diminishing amount of sex that bothers them, but its increasing dullness. They like to be proactive, and they're shopping for new tools.

I can think of a number of things that I could suggest to this couple, joining them in their practical approach to the problem of diminishing desire. But I question the rationalist approach in matters of the heart. I think that the challenge of sustaining eros in a committed relationship over time is of a different nature. We don't always know our aims in advance. Our desires are not exempt from conflict; nor are our passions free of contradictions. No amount of will or reason can dictate our love dreams. Reason doesn't know the roots of our dreams; nor does it know the mysterious needs of the heart. We can't always use the laws of profit and loss in our romantic and erotic lives. Applying the work ethos is tricky. Even the most logical approach cannot neutralize the ambivalence of love.

I tell Ryan and Christine, "I have nothing new to offer in the 'how to' department. You've had dates, you've been burning incense, you've cracked into the Astroglide. And it's landed you a steady diet of sex that's satisfactory without being really satisfying. Do I get it?"

"Yes, you get it, but what are you saying? That that's it? Like the song, 'Is That All There Is?'" Christine asks.

"There's no logic to this. Passion is unpredictable; it doesn't follow the dictates of cause and effect. What works on Monday might not work on Thursday. The solution is often a surprise, not the result of the kind of work you've been doing until now. So let's not talk about work. Instead, let's talk about freedom. Play."

"Huh?"

"Try something with me," I suggest to them. "It may seem off the beaten path; but since your path has become a dead end, you may as well give it a shot. What rigidifies desire is confinement. I'd like you to think about its opposite: freedom. Talk about it in the broad sense. When do you feel most free in your relationship? In what ways does being married make you more free, and in what ways does it make you less free? How much freedom are you comfortable giving each other? Giving yourselves?" I start the conversation in my office in the hope that they'll continue it on their own.

I like to make suggestions that might jolt people out of their complacency, or at least bring about a different way of thinking. I try to create some discomfort with the status quo. Although Ryan and Christine are unhappy with their situation, I'm not sure if they're unhappy enough to brave change. In therapy I throw out a lot of ideas, never knowing where they'll land or if they'll take root. I let the idea of freedom sit for a while, to see if it will sprout.

A few months later Ryan begins one session by announcing: "All right, you want to hear a real midlife story? You're going to get one. My wife's best friend from college came to visit us recently. You know I work from home, so we've had lunch together a few times with the babysitter and the kids—definitely not a pickup scene." Barbara is a humanitarian worker in her mid-forties who runs programs in crisis situations all over the world. No kids, a serial monogamist, independent, she's committed to the cause but getting a little tired of the lifestyle. He goes on, "She's beautiful, too, did I mention that? She lives the life I didn't live. I feel middle-age and middle-class around her. Nothing wrong with that, you'll say, but her adrenaline is contagious. She really hits a nerve in me, and she excites me. I've developed this amazing crush on her. You know how I've been talking about this feeling of deadness, my energy dropping, my body getting heavier? It's like when I settled down, I shut down. Well, her energy has woken me up. I want to kiss her. I'm scared to do it and scared not to. I feel like a fool, guilty, but I can't stop thinking about her. You know, I meant it when I made my vows. I'm in love with my wife; this has nothing to do with her. It's about something I've lost that I'm afraid I'll never get back."

When Ryan married Christine, he slammed the door on cruising. He left his struggling acting career, turned his paralegal moonlighting into a full-time job, and applied for law school. Now he works for environmental organizations as a legal consultant. As I listen to him sounding bewildered by his crush, I see an awakening of his dormant senses. I don't discourage Ryan's "immature" wishes, and I don't lecture him. Nor do I try to talk reason into him or explore the emotional dynamics beneath this presumably "adolescent" crush. I simply value his experience. He is looking at something beautiful; fantasizing about Barbara is a way of living the life he hasn't chosen. I marvel with him at the allure of the enchantment, while also calling it by its true name: a fantasy. The question I pose to him is how he can relish this experience without allowing the momentary exhilaration to endanger his marriage.

"How beautiful and how pathetic," I say. "It's great to know you can still come to life like that. And you know that you can never compare this state of intoxication with life at home, because home is about something else. Home is safe. Here, you're trembling; you're on shaky ground. You like it, but you're also afraid that it can take you too far away. I think that you probably don't let your wife evoke such tremors in you. There's an evolutionary anthropologist named Helen Fisher who explains that lust is metabolically expensive. It's hard to sustain after the evolutionary payoff: the kids. You become so focused on the incessant demands of daily life that you short-circuit any electric charge between you.

At our next session, Ryan knows exactly where he wants to start. Earlier that week, Christine and Barbara had made plans to go out to dinner. Feeling guilty, as she usually does, about going out without him, Christine invited Ryan to come along. Then she proceeded to ignore him for the rest of the evening. For once, he didn't mind taking a backseat as he watched the women reminisce. After college they had both spent a year in Togo with the Peace Corps. Christine came home; Barbara never did. As was often the case in their conversations, each reported her envy of and admiration for the life of the other.

"We'd just finished a great bottle of Australian Shiraz," said Ryan, "and we were all pretty tipsy, when Christine totally shocked me by blurting out to Barbara, 'I look at you and I wonder if it's worth it. Frankly, I don't think I'm made for this—the kids, the house, the job. Sometimes I wonder if I did it just to prove I could.' Then she says, 'I find it all so oppressive.' She wondered if it was all worth it—she finds it oppressive? I was stunned." Ryan repeated these words in a dazed voice as if he still couldn't quite believe hearing them. At my prodding, he told me the rest of his wife's remarks—that she felt she had always just done what was expected of her, that this was easier than figuring things out on her own. He continued, his tone both mocking and full of admiration as he expertly mimicked his wife. " 'I know it's not right to complain when you have it all,' she says. 'Where's my gratitude? I'm blessed with the kids, with Ryan, the remnants of a decent career, good friends. When you don't have it—the family, the marriage—you romanticize it. At least I did. But then when you do have it, you feel trapped. I have my blissful moments, but mostly I'm mired in drudgery.'"

Ryan said nothing at the time, but he was shocked. "How was I supposed to know she felt that way? She always looked happy enough to me. I thought she had what she wanted. I thought I was the only one feeling restless." Now, he was divided. On one hand he was angry that she hadn't lived up to his expectations; on the other, he was anxious about what her polemic said about him. "In my mind, she's a rock, I'm the squirmy one. I've had to work hard at being who I thought she wanted me to be, creating this life together. I felt put down. If she feels trapped, mired in drudgery, what does that make me?"

"Do you need her to acknowledge your hard work?" I asked.

"I guess so. Somehow her doubts diminished the value of my efforts. But then, this weird thing happened." He paused before speaking again. "I started to like it."

"Explain," I said.

"It's like I did a complete 180. I couldn't interrupt her, which I probably would have done if we'd been alone—not that she would ever say this stuff to me, anyway. Besides, I was intrigued. She felt just like I did; she was saying the very same things I didn't dare say. She wanted more. She was hungry, too. She missed her freedom. She kept becoming more interesting to me, more foreign. The wine really loosened her tongue."

"What else did she say?" I, too, was curious. The actor in him couldn't resist playing her part.

"'I feel like we're just stuck together,'" he said, again imitating her voice. "'Sometimes I fantasize about other lives, other men. Not any one man in particular—I just imagine a clean slate, unencumbered, no history, no problems. Someone I could be different with. I get so resentful that I am stuck in this house, in this family, inside my body. All I want to say is leave me alone, don't bother me.'"

Ryan shared with me the unexpected denouement of the evening. "I started out shocked and then defensive and then angry. But, weirdly, the more she was going on and on, the more I wanted her. She was on fire. At first I thought, oh, just quit the diatribe; but then I was captivated by her, I identified with her, and in a strange way I felt closer to her and more turned on than I had in a long time. My fascination with Barbara vanished. And I knew that if I'd married Barbara I'd be longing for Christine."

"And you didn't have to work for it," I say. "I couldn't have sent you home with an assignment that would have had this kind of result." I explain to him that his renewed desire came from her reassertion of her separateness and her dreams. When she voiced her unrequited longings, she gave Ryan permission to unleash his.

It's all highly impractical sometimes. The same scenario with a different couple might have triggered a fear of abandonment that would have caused the fight of the century. Nobody can plan for this; that's the point. Desire is an enigma; it's insubordinate, and it chafes at impositions. That evening, Ryan was receptive to Christine. In her honesty, he discovered her again. Even more important, he was choosing her again, and it's the act of choosing, the freedom involved in choosing, that keeps a relationship alive.

The flambé that Ryan and Christine savored that night had nothing efficient or expedient to it. It wasn't a task they could incorporate into their weekly routine. Christine rattled the cage, and Ryan was dislodged. She claimed her individuality, and the end result was greater intimacy. Desire emerged from a paradox: mutually recognizing the limitations of married life created a bond between them; acknowledging otherness inspired closeness.

There is no way to "institutionalize" or create a personal marital policy for this couple that will somehow ensure that they will go on having, or ever again have, this experience. As a therapist I acknowledge that setting up some kind of programmatic reinforcement to help them maintain this newfound glow is beyond my ability. But even though I can't turn this into an assignment or exercise, the fact that it happened may wake them up to a different kind of reality. It's my hope that it will change the way they look at themselves and each other.

"A Paradox to Manage, Not a Problem to Solve"

What makes sustaining desire over time so difficult is that it requires reconciling two opposing forces: freedom and commitment. So it's not only a psychological or practical problem; it's also a systemic one. That makes it harder to "work at." It belongs to the category of existential dilemmas that are as unsolvable as they are unavoidable. Ironically, even the business world, which is all about pragmatism and effectiveness, recognizes that some problems do not have clear solutions.

We find the same polarities in every system: stability and change, passion and reason, personal interest and collective well-being, action and reflection (to name but a few). These tensions exist in individuals, in couples, and in large organizations. They express dynamics that are part of the very nature of reality. Barry Johnson, an expert on leadership who is the author of *Polarity Management: Identifying and Managing Unsolvable Problems*, describes polarities as sets of interdependent opposites that belong to the same whole—you can't choose one over the other; the system needs both to survive.

Ben, for example, has a new girlfriend every six months, and each time he's convinced he's found "the one." But when the erotic intensity wanes even slightly, he panics and bails, thinking, "It's all downhill from here. I guess it wasn't love after all." He talks a lot about wanting a stable relationship—he wants commitment, he's ready to pair up—but his tolerance for sexual ennui is nil. In Ben's experience, commitment and excitement are mutually exclusive.

But in his fantasy, there is an omnipotent woman out there who can make it all come together. Her enchanting powers will ensure that the sex remains vibrant—the clearest sign of enduring love. She will be a woman who is so extraordinary, so amazing, that her sheer perfection will induce him to want to settle down (as if all this has nothing to do with him). Invariably, her unavailability is her single most attractive feature. He's been saying the same thing for years, "I just haven't found the right person yet. I've met loads of women. I just haven't met the right one, the one I could really stay with. I ask my friends who they would set me up with, and they can't think of anyone either. So you see?" Ben is in perpetual search for the ideal woman. Of course, he's been looking for a long time: even the most idealized creature ultimately turns out to be merely human, and therefore flawed.

At the beginning of each encounter he is swept away, and free from his inner turmoil. Invariably, when the initial ascent levels of, his phantoms reappear, as even the most beautiful princess will not deliver him from himself, or from the challenges of love. No matter how extraordinary she is, she can't protect him from the tedium that comes with time and its disillusionments. After each failed relationship he falls into what Octavio Paz calls a "swamp of concupiscence"—what we more commonly refer to as a sex binge. These multiple encounters offer him Olympian pleasures at night, but only sea-level dialogue the next morning. So each encounter quickly starts to feel empty, and he again finds himself yearning for the fantasy of connection with a stable partner. Hungry after months of casual sex, he approaches his new conquest with no less panic. Every time Ben falls in love, he goes from zero to 100 in one swoop. He can't pace himself. He can't get enough. He incorporates her, and not just sexually. It's the opposite swing of the pendulum—totally symmetrical and just as intense.

People like Ben are easily disparaged for their extreme reactions, but they're also a compelling topic of conversation. Ben is the one people like to gossip about with a mixture of pity (mainly the women) and envy (mainly the men). He's a live version of the conflict that so many of us experience silently, or in a more subdued fashion.

Knowing Ben's romantic nature, I'm reluctant to prescribe concrete sexual interventions designed to recharge his libido. Ben is advice-resistant; pragmatic solutions don't work for him, because his quandary is less something to repair than something to acknowledge. With this in mind, I borrow an exercise from Barry Johnson. I tell Ben, "I want you to breathe in and keep the air in as long as you can." Fresh oxygen inevitably turns into suffocating carbon dioxide, forcing him to exhale. At first, the release feels wonderful, but a few moments later he craves fresh oxygen again. I explain, "You can't choose between inhaling and exhaling; you have to do both. It's the same thing with intimacy and passion." I explain to Ben that the tension between security and adventure is a paradox to manage, not a problem to solve. It is a puzzle. "Can you hold the awareness of each polarity? You need each at different times, but you can't have both at the same time. Can you accept that? It's not an either-or situation, but one where you get the benefits of each and also recognize the limits of each. It's an ebb and flow." Love and desire are two rhythmic yet clashing forces that are always in a state of flux and always looking for the balance point.

Ben has been going out with Adair for the past eight months—a record for him—and something different is happening. "I think I'm in love with this woman," he says. "OK, I think I'm in love with every woman, but this one is different. OK, everyone is different, but this one is really different. She grounds me. I can be freaking out about something—you know how I get—and she doesn't react. Not that she doesn't care, or doesn't respond, but she doesn't get in there and panic right along with me. There's something quiet about her, and, you know, I'm anything but quiet. I think this could work. I like being with her. And the sex is still pretty good . . ."

"I'm waiting for the but . . ." I tell him.

"But I do feel it changing. I'm getting nervous, restless. I really don't want to fuck this up. I'm forty-three-years old, for God's sake. I want to have a kid, but I'm afraid I won't be able to stick around."

I have never met Adair, but something about the way she handles Ben makes me feel optimistic. Unbeknownst to him, he has a foil for his (dare I say?) fear of intimacy. In the past his girlfriends have been only too happy to merge with him; but Adair is able to hold her own—she seems to have a real sense of self that exists independently of him. Even after eight months, she is fiercely discreet about her private life. She exudes a quiet equanimity, a sober and subtle intelligence. She is a nurse in a pediatric oncology unit and works in the looming presence of death. Ben makes her laugh; he brings lightness into her world. His thirst for life enlivens her. His erotic ardor is the opposite of morbid. She likes the contrast.

Ben certainly brings an entire emotional history to his predicament, and he's got a lot of stuff to deal with. But the difficulty of reconciling security and excitement is not purely the result of his personal problems. It is the challenge of the modern ideal of love. With this in mind, we examine what sexuality means for Ben.

Most of us lament the wilting of erotic passion with melancholy, quiet acquiescence, or severe agita; but maintaining erotic vitality doesn't become the organizing principle of our lives. Not so for Ben. Sex is where he finds himself most alive. It has a regenerative power that allows him to go back into the world feeling enriched and renewed. In lovemaking he feels connection and nurturance that he does not get anywhere else. He is at once vulnerable and masterful, exposed and confident. Ben is a man with an active brain. Subjected to high-octane libidinal impulses, he's driven mostly in high gear. He gets frantic and disorganized, yet his hyperactivity has served him well in running his own courier company. For Ben, sex is the ultimate regulatory experience that quells his manic energy: extreme tension is followed by total release. At no other time does he feel as calm as when he has reached the hedonistic apex. It's a moment of perfect harmony between him and the world. And while Adair likes sex, Ben needs it. Sex is his life support—unplug it and he thinks he's dying. No wonder he panics at the thought of sex going downhill.

Ben is a modern man par excellence. He is action-driven, and that is why his typical response to sexual restlessness is to end the relationship, start going out again, have hot sex with someone else, and start a new relationship that will, he hopes, be inoculated against erotic demise. I point out to Ben that, contrary to popular belief, taking action is not always the best course.

"The first thing is not to act instantly on your panic and shut Adair out as a way to get rid of your anxiety," I tell him. "Less sex doesn't necessarily mean less love." I offer a safe container for his stirred-up anxiety, and I encourage him to think through the contradictions of desire rather than act them out. This pushes Ben out of his old way of thinking. I ask him to acknowledge his dilemma and to observe it with compassion and lucidity. Working through a conflict is not the same as eliminating it. In the recognition and management of the duality lies the survival of desire.

For Ben, acting out sexually is a short-lived solution. It provides a temporary salve to his anxiety, allowing him to duck the harder questions: What would it take for him to feel excited and safe in the same relationship? Why are exhilaration and playfulness cordoned off from love and commitment in his mind? How can he preserve a sense of freedom in the midst of an intimate relationship?

I reinterpret Ben's anxiety by suggesting that it can serve him as an early-warning system against complacency. "In the past, you reacted to your anxiety by bolting. I want you to think of it as a tool instead. Your anxiety is your ally, a barometer of your need to take some risks. When you start to feel antsy, it's time for something—not someone—new." I give him the following quotation from Frank Jude Boccio, author of *Mindfulness Yoga*, to think about as he leaves the session: "We bitch about our difficulties along the rough surface of our path, we curse every sharp stone underneath, until at some point in our maturation, we finally look down to see that they are diamonds."

We live in times where faster is better and control is power, where performance trumps process and risk is mathematically calculated. In our overcommitted lives there's a temptation to simplify our existential complexities. We just don't have the time and patience for open-ended reflection. We prefer instead to be proactive and thereby reaffirm our sense of control. In my practice I meet couples who complain about how the routine of their lives has left them feeling numb. But when we continuously invest in the kind of pragmatic solutions for "doing sex" that promise regularity—a decent average—we run the risk of exacerbating the blandness we struggle to remedy. Eroticism challenges us to seek a different kind of resolution, to surrender to the unknown and ungraspable, and to breach the confines of the rational world.

6

Sex Is Dirty; Save It for Someone You Love
When Puritanism and Hedonism Collide

Sex without sin is like an egg without salt.

—*Luis Buñuel*

I regret to say that we of the FBI are powerless to act in cases of oral-genital intimacy, unless it has in some way obstructed interstate commerce.

—*J. Edgar Hoover*

WHY DO SO MANY COUPLES become erotically alienated? The list of factors that contribute to the waning of excitement is long, and the one most commonly invoked is stress. "As soon as I sit down, I see the laundry that still needs folding, the unopened mail, the strewn toys, and it takes all sexual desire away from me." "Between our new jobs, our old parents, and our young kids, I'm wiped out. I don't have a very strong sex drive to begin with, but right now I don't have any desire for it at all. Don't take it personally." But when my patients cite the all-too-real stresses of modern life to explain why romance went south, I suggest that there may be more to it. After all, stress was a reliable feature of their lives long before they met, and it didn't stop them from leaping into one another's arms.

In the next tier of justification they trot out the deeper problems in the relationship: the heated bickering and icy standoffs, the lack of trust, the chronic disappointments, the cycles of blame. "Sex? You must be kidding. After what you just said to me?" "When's the last time you showed me you were interested?" "Do you think you could put just a little effort into making yourself attractive?" "I wish you'd shut the damned TV off; it makes me feel like dead meat."

This litany of disenchantment notwithstanding, I believe there's an additional layer to our libidinal demise that has to do with our culture's deep ambivalence around sexuality. While we recognize the importance of sex, we nonetheless vacillate between extremes of excessive license and repressive tactics: "Don't do it till you're married." "Just do it when you feel like it." "It's no big deal." "It's a huge deal." "You need love." "What's love got to do with it?" It's an all-or-nothing approach to sex. Porn sites proliferate on the Internet, yet we continue to debate whether or not to provide sex education in our schools and, if so, whether we should call it "Sex Ed" or opt for the less graphic "Health Ed."

Despite living in a time of unprecedented sexual freedom in America, the practice of policing sexuality has continued unabated since the days of the Puritans. State intervention makes some of us breathe a sigh of relief while leaving others stricken with terror. We promote abstinence with fear-based tactics, threaten straying politicians with impeachment, fight gay marriage, and gnaw away at the fragile abortion laws. Though virginity seems a relic of a bygone era, every day our elected officials bring moral gravitas to the legislation of sexuality. Abortion, homosexuality, adultery, and "family values" have been active items on the national political agenda for more than thirty years. This sexual conservatism is rooted in the Puritan tradition, with its deep suspicion of pleasure and its moralistic attitude toward anything that strays from hetero-sexual, monogamous, marital, reproductive sexuality.

Meanwhile, television producers invite us to phone in if we've had more than 100 sexual partners. Never before has sex been so publicly displayed, an incessant barrage of explicit images wher-ever we rest our eyes. Sex, the perennial default for advertising, has also become a commodity in itself. Tune in to almost any daytime talk show to hear about mothers who sleep with their daughters' boyfriends, men who like to watch, and housewife prostitutes who come out to their unsuspecting husbands. Sex is everywhere, in all its permutations, as exhaustively described by Lillian Rubin: "por-nography, impotence, premarital sex, marital sex, extramarital sex, group sex, swinging, S-M, and as many of the other variations of sexual behavior their producer can think of, whether the ordinary or the bizarre."

The politics and economics of sex and the diametrically opposed attitudes we witness daily penetrate the American bedroom and insinuate themselves into the creases of our intimacy. The couples I see live at the intersection of this ambivalence, and must negoti-ate amid these competing value systems. The legacy of Puritanism, which locates the family at the center of society, expects marriage to be reasonable, sober, and productive. You work, you save, and you plan. You take your commitments seriously. But alongside this very American notion of individual responsibility and moderation is the equally apple-pie notion of individual freedom. We believe in personal fulfillment: in life, liberty, and the pursuit of happiness. We relish the freedom to spontaneously satisfy our desires, and we live in a market-driven consumer economy which ensures that those desires never stop coming. The sexual culture tells us what is attractive and what we should want (as if we were incapable of finding out for ourselves whom to desire and what turns us on). An entire industry of hedonism hovers on the outskirts of marriage, a constant reminder of all we've sacrificed in exchange for the muted sexuality of marital love.

Can our modern-day relationships ever be strong enough to withstand the siren song of unlimited pleasure? When we are constantly exhorted to replace the old with the new, when sexual images forever portray youth and beauty (since nobody ages but you), when online sex caters to your most idiosyncratic whim, can we reasonably expect to remain contented with the same person for fifty years? The jury is still out. We're promised immediate fulfillment, and it's there for the taking by everyone but us. And all this reinforces the profound disconnect between what we're encouraged to want and what we're allowed to have. Puritanism and hedonism collide.

"Not Me, Not Now" Versus "Safe Sex or No Sex"

Let's not be fooled into thinking that this saturation reflects enlightened sexual attitudes. The blatant marketing of sexual images may be more excessive than progressive, and it has at its roots profit and the freedom of the market rather than freedom of thought. In short, it's more about opening your wallet than opening your mind. Perhaps this is why our culture's underlying "city on a hill" morality remains unsoiled by all the graphic images that flicker on our screens: the central idea that sex is dirty remains unchallenged.

Nowhere is our profound discomfort with sex more apparent than in the way we approach teenage sexuality. A sizable group of Americans believe that limiting access to birth control and sex education will steer our teenagers away from the temptations of the flesh. Campaigns like "Not Me, Not Now" encourage abstinence as a means of avoiding teen pregnancy and sexually transmitted diseases, and our public health policies reflect the idea that adolescent sexuality is deviant behavior that should be prevented. No matter how liberated the media may appear, to many Americans sexuality is considered deeply dangerous—a risk factor.

Europeans, in contrast, view adolescent sexuality as a normal developmental stage on the way to healthy adult sexuality. Sex is not a problem; being irresponsible about sex is. Hence the European counter-slogan to "Not Me, Not Now" is "Safe Sex or No Sex." It's also worth noting that in Europe, teenagers engage in sexual activity an average of two years later than their American counterparts, and the rate at which teenagers give birth is a staggering eight times less. How is it that American society, with such a clear bias against teen sex, produces such a statistical embarrassment?

Taboo-ridden sexuality and excess-driven sexuality converge in a troubling way. Both lead us to want to dissociate psychically from the physical act of sex. A society that sees sex as soiled does not make sex go away. Instead, this kind of anxious atmosphere breeds guilt and shame in its more extreme version, or a generalized discomfort in its more ubiquitous expression. Sex is divorced from emotional and social continuity. What is missing is a sexuality that is integrated, in which pleasure flourishes in a context of relatedness. I'm not talking only about deep love; I'm also talking about basic care and appreciation for another person.

Want to Hook Up Tonight?

Ratu is a twenty-two-year-old college student at an Ivy League university. She is the daughter of a doctor and a computer programmer, both Indian immigrants, whose years of hard work have paid off in an upmarket lifestyle. Ratu spent twelve years in the highly competitive public schools of New York City, and now hopes to follow her mother into medicine. I met Ratu's mother at a friend's going-away party. When I told her the subject of my book, she urged me to interview her daughter. "What I hear from my daughter? It is just unbelievable. So bleak, the way these children treat each other. You really want to know what is going on? You should talk to her. I cannot get my head around it."

I knew I had to meet Ratu, and I did. Bright and articulate, she was like a spokesperson for one of those generations with a letter attached to it—X or Y or whatever they're up to now. She gave me an illuminating description of the sexual scene on campus.

"We don't really have time to date. So the quick fix is the Friday or Saturday night hookup. You go to a party or you go to a bar; everyone gets drunk, really drunk, and everyone pairs off. It's over and done with by the time Monday rolls around, after everyone has shared hookup stories over lunch. 'Hookup' is sort of a broad term that covers everything from just fooling around to oral sex to full-on sex.

"The ideal college relationship is the 'friends-with-benefits' scenario. You have a close male friend who you have a lot of fun with and with whom there is a bit of sexual tension. It starts one night when you're both drunk and run into each other at a bar or something. You go home together, have sex (great or not so great, it doesn't matter) and then pretend it didn't happen. The next week this is repeated with the same person, and so on and so forth, until you feel as though you don't need the pretense of going out and getting drunk. Instead you just call him when you feel like hooking up or if you're just bored."

This is what Ratu and her friends unapologetically refer to as the booty call. There is an emotional downside, even to this stunningly abbreviated form of coupling. "There comes a point," Ratu says, "when one party gets more involved than the other and it's time for the uncomfortable talk. Ground rules are established: this is simply a friends-with-benefits scenario, nothing more, nothing less; and if he or she isn't OK with that, then it's over. And then you move on to another friend. We try very hard not to let our emotions get in the way," says Ratu without a trace of irony.

What's interesting for me in Ratu's description is that there's no arc to this narrative—no ascending plot, no unfolding, no climax, no closure. In fact, there's no *story* to the story at all. Sex is separated from the story that brought it into being. "There is a deliberate attempt to keep emotions out of sex, and not just for the boys," Ratu elaborates. "The girls as well as the boys speak of love on one hand and sex on the other, as though they have nothing to do with each other." She pauses, "Though I suspect that a lot of my girlfriends would rather be in relationships, whether or not they want to admit it."

Far be it from me to disparage the liberating expression of casual or recreational sex. An erotic encounter can span a range of interpersonal intensities without being disaffiliated. But this particular type of sexual activity seems less an expression of liberation than an acting out of underlying anxiety. To my surprise, Ratu agreed with this idea completely. "The drinking and the sex, of course they go together. They're both things we know we're not supposed to be doing."

As I listened to Ratu, I wondered how this new sociology of sex would manifest itself later in their committed relationships. "What about love and marriage?" I asked her. "Does that ever come up?"

"We see commitment as a life sentence. I know especially for many of my male friends it's a terrifying thought. They can't imagine having the same sexual partner for more than a week, let alone ten years." Then Ratu says more seriously, "For the women it's different. They can see the appeal. Some really seem to want it, though a lot of us take on the stereotypical male fear and see monogamy as a restriction. Commitment means sacrificing your own goals and ambitions for something that you can't control and that you could potentially fail at. At least that's how we think of it now. Relationships are a loss of independence. When you let another person in, romantically, you make less room for yourself."

"So relationships are about what you lose, not what you gain?" I ask.

"Exactly."

"And romance?"

"Hah. There was none in high school. The few couples here at college stand out as almost weird, like they're married or something."

I am intrigued by Ratu's portrayal of relationships. It had always seemed to me that coupling (or at least the dream of romance) enlarges us, and is about what you can discover with someone. At least, I was convinced of that at her age. Ratu and her friends seem to find more security in an MBA than in the power of a sustaining, loving bond. Why do they feel this way?

One reason might be that having embraced the cultural mandate of self-reliance, they are apprehensive about relationships. "If you add love to sex you make yourself extremely vulnerable," she tells me. "I think that might be the heart of the issue for my whole generation, this lack of trust. We were taught to rely on ourselves, not to depend on others." It's an unromantic attitude, but perhaps a wise one, given the precariousness of modern marriage. Gender equality is made manifest in all its irony: both men and women now have the right to be terrified of commitment. Better to engage in risky sex than to succumb to the risks of the heart.

Nothing is more useless than predicting the future for someone who's not interested in hearing it; but sometimes I can't resist, so I ventured an insight with Ratu. "You're making me think that maybe this is why so many of the couples I see have such a hard time having hot sex with the one they love. It's not just your generation. This entire culture is profoundly uncomfortable with vulnerability and dependency. Good intimate sex requires both."

"Maybe," Ratu says. "But who said good sex has to be intimate? What if 'good' means throw me against the wall, ravish me, and leave before I wake up in the morning? It's the spontaneity I love. It's the excitement that comes with the spontaneity and the multiple partners and the dream dates where nothing goes wrong because after brunch the next day you say good-bye and don't stick around long enough to see each other's flaws. I go through periods of being addicted to that excitement, but I also go through periods when I recognize how superficial it all is and I want a deeper connection with someone. I have had boyfriends, and it's nice, though it does get a little boring. Hopefully somewhere in there I'll find a healthy balance—if I haven't already spoiled myself to the point of dissatisfaction with long-term relationships."

Far from being the last word on free love, all this bravado belies an underlying unease. I wonder to what extent this kind of hit-and-run sex is actually a defense against sexual discomfort, in much the same way that taboo-ridden avoidance is a defense. It's the flip side of the coin: same anxiety, different response. They get drunk, have sex, then *pretend it never happened*. It's a way of doing it without being in it. It all just happens; no one has to own it. Perhaps these pretend libertines are not nearly as removed from the Puritan legacy as their Saturday night romps would lead us to believe. Their furtive encounters are not exactly a celebration of the pleasures of the flesh. If there wasn't at least a shred of moral dissonance in their desire for sex, they might not need to get hammered in order to have it. If they were more comfortable with sex, they would actually place themselves in the heart of it and would want to remember it.

For Ratu, the excitement born of spontaneity is ensured as long as she changes partners frequently enough. But what will happen to her when she's left with only one? I may never meet Ratu again, but many of the people who come to see me remind me of her. They have found that their history of sexual nomadism is no help in meeting the challenge of sustaining sexual vitality with one person over time. They view sex before marriage and sex after marriage as entirely different realities. Single sex isn't supposed to prepare you for committed sex. If anything, it's seen as the last hurrah before a lifetime of sexual decline.

How Important Is Sex Anyway?

A healthy sense of erotic entitlement is built on a relaxed, generous, and unencumbered attitude toward the pleasures of the body—something our puritan culture continues to grapple with. I witness the fallout of this ambivalence in my practice every day. Much of my work with couples involves addressing the shame and anxiety that surround people's sexuality, causing them to want to withdraw from their lovers for fear of being judged and rejected. I give permission, reduce anxiety, normalize fantasies and desires, and challenge the distortions of poor body image. Together we excavate the secrets and the silence that accompanied their sexual upbringing, and confront the cultural and familial messages that block erotic expression. Therapy is a process of expanding sexuality by shedding inhibitions, encouraging physicality, and negotiating boundaries. Couples learn to dance step by step, and it takes as long as it takes.

I met Maria when she was at the tail end of a heartbreak. She'd just spent two years on the west coast with a man she thought she was going to marry, only to come home a disillusioned wreck. Her friends decided it was time for her to meet a nice man, a mensch. Enough of these himbos (for those of you unfamiliar with this new term, himbos are male bimbos sought by successful women). The friends organized a dinner party with a mission: a tasteful cover-up for a first date. It worked.

For Maria, dating Nico was a reeducation in the art of love, a slow unfolding that was remarkably worry-free. She didn't fall in love; she grew to love him. But a year after meeting him, she's in my office, asking, "How important is sex, anyway? I keep going back and forth. I know you can't build a life on passion. I've tried that. My grandma used to say, 'What are you going to live on, love? Hah! You've got a lot to learn.' My mother's no better. Her line is, 'Sweetheart, passion is doomed. Take my word for it, what you need is to find someone you can live with. Someone who's like you, who shares your values. You know, money doesn't hurt, either.' I love Nico. I've never felt so secure, so trusting. And after years of being out there dating more than my share of jerks, I'm finally free to think about other things in my life. But I just don't know. I don't think we click sexually. It's an issue. Or is it? Everyone says that the sex fades anyway, no matter how steamy it is in the beginning, so how important is it, really?"

"You tell me," I prompt her.

"You know what I tell myself? 'Girl, you had your fun. It's time to grow up. He's a great guy. Get over yourself.'"

Three years after Maria asked me the question, "How important is sex, anyway?" she's back again. Evidently, she hasn't yet found her answer. In the beginning she was so taken up by the thrill of security that she was able to postpone dealing with her lack of sexual responsiveness to Nico. She held out some hope that the problem would take care of itself, that one day the block would lift and everything would fall into place. Nico, for his part, is a patient man. He wasn't going to push, even though he is clearly less than jolly about their anemic sex life. Not pushing the issue is his way of forestalling rejection. In our sessions Maria had always displayed an approach-avoidance attitude to the topic of sex. On the few occasions that she brought it up directly, it was always at the end of the hour, when there was no time left for discussion. One week I decided to keep my foot on the gas and rev up the conversation.

"Sex is hard, isn't it?" I asked her.

"What do you mean? Hard to talk about or hard to do?" she answered my question with a question.

"Hard to own." I replied.

"It's easier for me to have sex than to talk about it."

"And with Nico?"

"With Nico it's easier not to have sex than to talk about it."

"Tell me."

"Sex *is* hard. I don't want it a lot of the time, which is strange because I've always thought of myself as a sexual person. I read about women with low desire and I don't identify with them, even though it sounds like me lately."

"Was it easier with other men?"

"Oh, God, no—but in the past I never had to talk about it. It was never something I had to work on. Either it came naturally and we clicked, or the relationship wasn't going to last anyway, so why bother? Now I'm with a man I love. I think he's beautiful, he treats me like a queen, and I don't want to have sex with him. He gets frustrated when I reject him day after day, and I don't like the fact that I'm so indifferent to sex. I'd like to think it happened when I got pregnant with our daughter, but to be honest I was kind of relieved to have an excuse. 'I'm pregnant' turned into 'I just had a baby' turned into 'I'm nursing' turned into 'I need my sleep.' Truthfully, as you know, it's been a problem from the beginning."

"Shall we take the plunge?"

"I'm tired of avoiding it, of waiting for something to change. I can't swap Nico for a new model. I make it work with him or I shrivel up."

Maria grew up in a working-class family, the daughter of a policeman and a substitute teacher. Religion was central, and she attended all-girl Catholic schools through high school. "We never talked about sex at home. My grandma had ten kids and never knew women could have orgasms. Can you imagine? I haven't seen my mother naked since I was three. I've never seen my father naked. I'm the youngest of five, and each of us rebelled in our own way—though my brothers never had to face the injunctions reserved for the girls."

Maria sheds light on the pervasive all-or-nothing, feast or famine sexual culture in America. "I was seventeen when I lost my virginity; and for Catholic girls, once you've slept with one person you might as well sleep with the whole town—and, frankly, most of us did." she tells me. "I know it sounds archaic, but it really was like that where I grew up. Staten Island is like a nature preserve for endangered Catholics. The message was clear: sex is a sin unless you're married."

"Right. Like the old adage, 'Sex is dirty; save it for someone you love,'" I say.

Maria moved away, went to college, became a casting agent, and today lives in a world vastly different from that of her childhood. But all this intellectual broadening has not succeeded in dismantling the prohibitions: carnal lust is sinful, and especially for women. Despite twenty years of brief encounters, seasonal relationships, and steady boyfriends, the vestigial messages cling obstinately to the sinews of her body with a subcutaneous tenacity. Acting liberated doesn't necessarily mean being liberated. When she was still single, Maria could circumvent her latent sexual uneasiness. It was easier to be uninhibited when she had less invested emotionally. But once she chose to live within the geographic limitations of a family, the murmurs of her past began to echo.

"Once every six months or so I'll bring it up with Nico. I'll say, 'Nico, our sex life sucks. We need to do something about it. I want you to read this book.' But he doesn't want to read a book. He hates those books. He'll say, 'It's not my thing. Let's just make some time to be together. The more sex you have, the more sex you have, right?' That's his stock answer."

"I've recommended books to you before, but in this instance it sounds like you're using them to hide behind. Why is it so hard for you to talk about yourself? To be your own advocate? What would happen if you said, 'Nico, I want to tell you about myself—what I think and feel about sex, about myself sexually?'"

"The whole subject is so emotionally overwhelming it makes me sleepy."

Maria was taught that nothing is free; everything must be earned. Privilege is for those who've never had to work hard, and it's morally suspect. The credo was: you sacrifice for the good of the family. Her reluctance to put herself forward is particularly strong in the sexual realm.

"It seems OK to ask for what you really need," I explain, "but to ask for something just because you want it or like it is selfish. Pleasure itself, unless you've earned it, is dubious. It also raises the question of how much you feel you deserve and are worthy of receiving—just because you're you. But eroticism is precisely that: it's pleasure for pleasure's sake, offered to you gratuitously by Nico."

Together, Maria and I work on cultivating a healthy sense of deserving that spans sitting down in the morning when she drinks her coffee, reading the paper while the kitchen is still dirty, and going out with her friends even if it means Nico has to spend two nights in a row taking care of the baby. She is to take a break from the idea that pleasure must be paid for, in advance, by the performance of duty. We chisel away at this complex system of fairness and merit, where everything has to be perfectly equitable in order to neutralize selfishness.

Maria has taken hold of this idea. "I think my 'low desire' is, more than anything else, related to my lack of ownership around sex and my conflict with pleasure, especially pleasure with my husband. I can't explain why I'm so uncomfortable opening myself up to Nico erotically. What I do know is that family is never where I've gone to get anything extra."

"Right. For you, family is about self-sacrifice, not enjoyment. But a healthy sense of entitlement is a prerequisite for erotic intimacy."

Only when Maria starts to look at what she brings to the erotic stalemate does Nico's contribution become apparent. She asks him some of the same questions we have hashed out in our sessions. "What does sex mean for you?" "How was sex treated in your family?" "What are the important events that shaped your sexuality?" "What would you like to experience most with me sexually, and what are you most afraid of?" They spark conversations that are provocative and inspiring, that focus on possibilities rather than on problems.

Maria learns that, for Nico, sex is both liberating and connecting, an eloquent mark of love. When she rebuffs him, he feels unloved. Nico is not a talker. Instead, he expresses caring by doing things: washing the dishes, shining her shoes, always keeping chocolate in the refrigerator. He makes sure that they get out of the house on the weekend, guilt-free (which Maria finds difficult), and don't get bogged down with interminable housekeeping. He is generous with his affection, both with Maria and with their daughter. But the caresses stop when the sex starts. While he likes sex, he's less in his element with seduction. "He's so eager to get to the *sex* part of sex, where he knows what he's doing, that he tends to gloss over the pursuit and the romance. The games, you know. I wind up feeling rushed. It takes Nico about two minutes to go from watching TV to being completely physically and emotionally ready to have intercourse. I need a slower buildup. And in my typical way of trying to take care of him, I don't want him to feel bad, so I try to get turned on really fast. It's a total fiasco."

For Nico, sex is a play in one act. For Maria it is a continuum of pleasures, a successive unfolding. The problem arises when they become trapped in a linear, goal-oriented focus on intercourse and orgasm that bypasses eroticism. In this setup she struggles with the idea that lingering is implicitly selfish and shamelessly greedy. Her lack of prerogative and lack of self-affirmation are met with Nico's hurriedness, which further reinforces her notion that she is not worthy of attention. Of course she wouldn't worry that she was taking too long if she thought he was into it. But for Nico slowness inspires a different kind of anxiety, a fear of inadequacy that he won't perform well enough.

I suggest to Maria that she and Nico liberate themselves from this task-oriented performance model of sexuality with its rigid requirements for mutual orgasm. It's a pass-fail approach that smacks of seriousness and takes much of the fun out of sex.

"Remember making out?" I ask her. "When's the last time you did that?"

"It's been years. You know, I remember in the very beginning we spent an evening making out, French-kissing on the boardwalk at Coney Island. It was amazing. We don't do that anymore."

"Well, then, there you go."

The intricacies of the dynamics between Maria and Nico are subtle, and this is true for most of the couples I meet. It's never just one thing or one partner. Maria says she wants to be seduced, yet she resists seeing Nico as seductive. "My relationship stands in the way of my attraction to him. Sometimes I'll look at him, like when he gets out of the shower or comes home from the gym, and I'll think, 'God, he's hot.' Why is he so attractive until I remember he's my husband?"

I explain to Maria that it's scary to be both erotically exposed and emotionally intimate with the same person, especially when you hold the belief that sex is somehow shameful. "There's a whole part of you that hasn't yet entered your relationship. In fact, the psychic energy involved in keeping it tucked away is enough to make you exhausted. No wonder you'd rather go to sleep than make love to your husband."

Like many of us, Maria grew up learning to hide her erotic reveries and idle daydreams. Keeping our pleasures secret is a central component of our sexual socialization. Maria recalls the shame of getting caught as a child in a delicious moment of erotic exploration, and the disgust on her mother's face as she said, "Stop that right now." Even those of us fortunate enough to have parents who recognized that sexual play feels good are still likely to remember with a wince the admonishment, "Keep it private." It is hard to bring out in the open that which we spent years trying to hide.

Not surprisingly, Maria struggles to bring into her relationship the erotic imaginings she was taught so early to suppress and defend against. Sensing Nico's receptivity, it is precisely what I encourage her to do—to own the wanting, and to believe herself worthy of being cooed over. At the same time I encourage her to bring to Nico a fresh curiosity. "It is too easy to encase him in the role of husband, with all the attendant domestic qualities, and then complain about a lack of desire. He has a whole interior geography and you're just hanging around in the same old neighborhood."

This is the challenge of sexual intimacy, of bringing home the erotic. It is the most fearsome of all intimacies because it is all-encompassing. It reaches the deepest places inside us, and involves disclosing aspects of ourselves that are invariably bound up with shame and guilt. It is scary, a whole new kind of nakedness, far more revealing than the sight of our nude bodies. When we express our erotic yearnings we risk humiliation and rejection, which are equally devastating. I have witnessed the painful scene when a person's preferences are condemned and labeled by his or her partner as perverse, deviant, and disgusting. It is no wonder that many of us prefer the security of workable sex as a shield against this harrowing scenario. We may be far from passion, but at least we feel normal. In the grand scheme of things, it's not a bad compromise. But then there are those who long to be known differently, to give themselves over and risk crossing that threshold. They muster the courage to confront the cultural prohibitions against sex—exuberant sex—at home. They hunger for full expression in the erotic realm, and resist the urge to withhold. For them sexual communion is far from dirty, but rather a sacred melding that puts us in touch with the divine.

Erotic intimacy is the revelation of our memories, wishes, fears, expectations, and struggles within a sexual relationship. When our innermost desires are revealed, and are met by our loved one with acceptance and validation, the shame dissolves. It is an experience of profound empowerment and self-affirmation for the heart, body, and soul. When we can be present for both love and sex, we transcend the battleground of Puritanism and hedonism.

7

Erotic Blueprints

Tell Me How You Were Loved, and I'll Tell You How You Make Love

Grown-ups never understand anything for themselves, and it is tiresome for children to be always and forever explaining things to them.

—*Antoine de Saint-Exupéry,* The Little Prince

So, like a forgotten fire, a childhood can always flare up again within us.

—*Gaston Bachelard*

A HOST OF INSTITUTIONS LOOK out for our best interest. Religion, government, medicine, education, the media, and pop culture all labor tirelessly to define and regulate the parameters of our sexual well-being. The incentives and prohibitions surrounding the voluptuousness of the body are the mother's milk of society. Much of what we learn about sex comes from the street, the movies, television, and school. But before any of these reach us, our family gets to us first. We are members of a society, but we're also the children of our parents. (This includes grandparents, stepparents, guardians, foster parents, and anyone else who is entrusted with our early well-being.) No history has a more lasting effect on our adult loves than the one we write with our primary caregivers.

The Archaeology of Desire

The psychology of our desire often lies buried in the details of our childhood, and digging through the early history of our lives uncovers its archaeology. We can trace back to where we learned to love and how. Did we learn to experience pleasure or not, to trust others or not, to receive or be denied? Were our parents monitoring our needs or were we expected to monitor theirs? Did we turn to them for protection, or did we flee them to protect ourselves? Were we rejected? Humiliated? Abandoned? Were we held? Rocked? Soothed? Did we learn not to expect too much, to hide when we are upset, to make eye contact? In our family, we sense when it's OK to thrive and when others might be hurt by our zest. We learn how to feel about our body, our gender, and our sexuality. And we learn a multitude of other lessons about who and how to be: to open up or to shut down, to sing or to whisper, to cry or to hide our tears, to dare or to be afraid.

All these experiences shape our beliefs about ourselves and our expectations for others. They are part of the dowry each man and woman brings to adult love. Part of this emotional scorecard is obvious and manifest, but much of it is unspoken, concealed even from ourselves.

Our sexual preferences arise from the thrills, challenges, and conflicts of our early life. How these bear on our threshold for closeness and pleasure is the object of our excavation. What turns you on and what turns you off? What draws you in? What leaves you cold? Why? How much closeness can you stand to feel? Can you tolerate pleasure with the one you love?

When Steven's father abandoned his mother, she picked up the pieces, devoted herself to caring for her children, and swore she would never let anyone hurt her like that again. An ER nurse, today she owns her home and has put three kids through college. Steven is filled with admiration and respect for his mother, and has spent much of his life guarding against becoming what he calls, "that asshole." Six years into his marriage to Rita, he finds himself avoiding her *démarches* and ducking her accusations about his sexual passivity. Behind his excuses, Steven is baffled by his lack of interest—and by his unreliable erections.

The more he loves and respects his wife, the harder it is for him to *fuck* her. In Steven's mind, emotional security requires a constant monitoring of any selfish or aggressive inclinations. This belief, which grew out of his love for his mother, has become part of his sexuality. The more he loves Rita and the more he depends on her, the greater his need for caution and the more inhibited he is sexually. He doesn't know how to experience the open range of lust in the context of emotional care. His unconscious is loyal to the past.

For Dylan, a retail manager in his twenties, emotional security feels altogether impossible, with or without sexual excitement. His mother, who died when he was twelve, was the emotional linchpin of their family. When his eyes filled with tears at her funeral, his father said to him, "I hope you're not going to fall apart on me." In order to stay close to his father he had to excise his entire emotional life. He explains, "All feelings were a sign of weakness in our house." The minute Dylan has feelings for someone he lashes out at himself with self-loathing, hoping to control his unbearable vulnerability. His solution? Twice a week he goes to the clubs to pick up men he will never know and who—more important—will never know him. In anonymous sex there are no feelings, and Dylan is protected from repeating the humiliations of his childhood. At the same time he gets to experience the delicious thrill of being wanted, being chosen by many at once.

One aspect of the erotic blueprint that illustrates the irrationality of our desire is that what excites us most often arises from our childhood hurts and frustrations. The sex therapist Jack Morin explains that the erotic imagination is ingenious in undoing, transforming, and redressing the traumas of the past. In other words, the experiences that caused us the most pain in childhood sometimes become the greatest sources of pleasure and excitement later on.

Let's take a look at Melinda. Her father is a philanderer. And while she empathizes with her mother's despair, she also doesn't want to be like her mother: broken, miserable, bereft. Instead she has become the seductress, the opposite of the abandoned wife. Melinda sets out to best men at their own game. Desire is stoked by unavailability in Melinda's mind, and once she's seduced a man he is instantly less attractive. In order to reconfirm her own power she must set her sights on the next man, and the next, and the next. If there is no obstacle to clear, she has no way to gauge her value. Almost nothing is more exciting than conquering a powerful, aloof man; but the ultimate thrill is in dumping him—sure proof that she has avenged the past. In heartlessly dismissing these men, Melinda seeks to confirm that, unlike her mother, she is strong and independent, the one calling the shots, making the choices, picking up or discarding lovers as suits her fancy. Of course, by ruthlessly purging vulnerability from her life, she perversely ends up just as lonely and unloved as her mother.

The central agent of eroticism is the human imagination, but for many people the project of sexual self-discovery is hampered by parental messages that induce fear, guilt, and mistrust. Something that is meant to protect children often turns out to be a source of much anxiety in adult sexual love. Lena grew up with a roster of what is and is not acceptable for a worthy woman to dream about, act on, and get off on. The eldest daughter in a conservative, devoutly religious household, Lena learned that decent women hewed to strict standards of womanly behavior, were never aggressive or pushy, and always put the needs of others before their own. Like her mother (and centuries of women before her) Lena has derived her self-esteem and validation from being a giver and not a taker. By making herself indispensable, she has hoped to counteract the vagaries of love. But Lena's niceness is precisely what turns her husband off. Her coy lovemaking and her lack of sexual assertiveness inhibit him.

In recent months Lena has started to wonder what her marriage would be like if she were less accommodating. She is experimenting with the idea that she might be liked for who she is, not only for what she gives. Together we have been deconstructing the anxiety, guilt, and self-abnegation that are the legacy of the nice girl. Lena would love to become bold enough not only to know what she likes but to be able to ask for it. Buying lingerie at Victoria's Secret with her husband may not sound like much, but for Lena it was as uplifting as a Wonderbra.

The internal tensions that crackle in the sexuality of Steven, Dylan, Melinda, and Lena are a result of childhood conflicts. The details of our erotic proclivities and apprehensions are refined throughout our lives but often originate in our childhood experiences, both good and not so good. Sometimes it takes a bit of psychological sleuthing to make sense of all this, but very little in one's erotic imagination is happenstance.

Me in the Context of We

Our physical and emotional dependence on our parents surpasses that of any other living species, in both magnitude and duration. It is so complete—and our need to feel safe is so profound—that we will do anything not to lose them. We will suppress our wishes and push our aggression underground. We will take the blame for abuse, submit to control, become self-reliant, and otherwise renounce our needs. In short, we'll apply a wide range of self-preservation tactics, all aimed at maintaining our primary bond.

Things get tricky when you consider that one of our greatest needs, developmentally speaking, is autonomy. From the moment we can crawl, we navigate the treacherous paths of separation in an attempt to balance our fundamental urge for connection with the urge to experience our own agency. We need our parents to take care of us, but we also need them to give us enough space to establish our freedom. We want them to hold us and we want them to let us go.

Throughout our lives we grapple with this interplay between dependence and independence. How artfully we reconcile these needs as adults depends greatly on how our parents reacted to the stubborn duality in our little selves. It's important to point out that our parents' behavior, what they actually do, is only one part of the situation. Another part is our interpretation of their actions. Each child brings an individual resilience to the lottery of life. What might feel good to one will feel overwhelming to another. Some of us may wish our parents had been more involved, while others may cringe at memories of their parents' scrutiny and intrusion. Every family has its preferred responses to expressions of dependency and autonomy—when they are rewarded and when they are thwarted. In the give-and-take with our parents we determine how much freedom we can safely experience, and how much our connections will require the subjugation of our needs. In the end we fashion a system of beliefs, fears, and expectations—some conscious, many unconscious—about how relationships work. We wrap these up in a tidy package and hand it to our beloved. It is a fair trade.

Not coincidentally, this entire emotional history plays itself out in the physicality of sex. The body is the purest, most primal tool we have for communicating. As Roland Barthes wrote, "What language conceals is said through my body. My body is a stubborn child; my language is a very civilized adult." The body is our mother tongue—our mediator with the world long before we speak our first words. From the moment we come into being, love flows from adult to child sensuously—and I dare say erotically as well.

Bodily sensations dominate our first awareness of our environment and our earliest interactions with our caregivers. The body is a memory bank for the sensual pleasures of the skin. How often do I hear men and women in my office implore each other, "Can you just hold me?" The soothing powers of a hug hold at forty no less than at five. The body is also a storage facility for the distress and the frustration we have endured, and the pain we have suffered. Cleverly, our bodies remember what our minds may have chosen to forget, both light and dark. Perhaps this is why our deepest fears and most persistent longings emerge in intimate sex: the immensity of our neediness, the fear of desertion, the terror of being engulfed, the yearning for omnipotence.

Erotic intimacy is an act of generosity and self-centeredness, of giving and taking. We need to be able to enter the body or the erotic space of another, without the terror that we will be swallowed and lose ourselves. At the same time we need to be able to enter inside ourselves, to surrender to self-absorption while in the other's presence, believing that the other will still be there when we return, that he or she won't feel rejected by our momentary absence. We need to be able to connect without the terror of obliteration, and we need to be able to experience our separateness without the terror of abandonment.

The Selfishness of Intimate Pleasures

I have always been interested in the people who are able to achieve balance between self and other on an emotional level but who repeatedly fail to achieve it physically. The threat of merging in the physical act of sex, and the ensuing loss of self, is so intense for these people that they defend against it either by shutting down sexually or by taking their desire elsewhere. The psychoanalyst Jessica Benjamin writes, "The child's struggle for autonomy takes place within the realm of the body and its pleasures." It is no different for the adult.

The first time James walked into my office, he sat down and said, "Stella and I have a very good marriage, but sex has always been a problem." James feels sexually inhibited with Stella, and their erotic misfit fills him with tension. Whatever initial excitement he may feel when Stella approaches him invariably turns into a preoccupation with his own performance. Will I stay hard? Will I come too soon? Will Stella have an orgasm? Sex becomes a race to the finish line—can he get there before he loses his erection? His ability to enjoy himself is massively curtailed by this narrow focus. He can't be playful, can't try out new things, because anything that strays from the routine might jeopardize his capacity to perform. These anxieties always have a ripple effect, and James's inhibitions have also stifled Stella. She senses his absence, laments his lack of attention, and has complained about it bitterly over the years.

"Tell me about your mother," I ask James.

"My mother? You don't waste a minute, do you? A few years ago I went to see a therapist, and she also wanted me to talk about my mother. It didn't change a thing. My wife is nothing like my mother."

"In due diligence I always go back to the source. I promise I won't tell you that you married your mother. But the first place we learn about love and relationships is in our original family. None of the others—friends, flings, teachers, lovers—can carry this kind of emotional resonance. So, tell me about your mother."

What emerges in our conversations is that James was keenly attuned to his mother's moods, and she was often lonely and sad.

She didn't like noise, didn't like messes, and got agitated when he and his sister were too boisterous. She was a good mother, but very tightly wound. "I always found it difficult to handle the specifications of her needs. She needed seventy-two things lined up to be OK." James's mother relied on him for support, company, and conversation. (She referred to his father as simply the Paycheck.) "When I was older and wanted to do things with my friends, I knew she was disappointed. She'd say, 'Have a good time' in a way that made it very hard for me to have a good time." James grew up torn between his desire not to displease his mother and his need to lead his own life. "Getting a scholarship to Stanford, clear across the country, was the best thing that could have happened to me. She couldn't deny me that opportunity. I left, but I took a lot of guilt with me."

The first time James set eyes on Stella, she was a vision. "Everything about her was graceful, vibrant, colorful. Here was a woman who was not afraid to stand out. She was all light." Stella was the antithesis of James's mother, and for the first time he was able to love a woman and not feel burdened with responsibility and guilt. In fact, Stella regularly rejected his attempts to be overly accommodating, explaining that they made her feel smothered. He laughs when he recounts how anxious he used to feel when he wanted to do something that didn't include her—he was always afraid of disappointing her. He had a way of asking, "Do you mind?" that drove her crazy. Finally she snapped, "Look, I'm not your mother. You don't have to ask my permission." Stella has taught James, largely through example, that you can be close to someone—intimate, caring, secure—without feeling sacrificed in the process. In asserting her independence, Stella has communicated over and over that she's not fragile, and that her well-being does not depend exclusively on him. The price of love does not have to be personal obliteration.

In many ways, James and Stella have an enviable marriage. They enjoy each other. He still makes her laugh out loud, and she is the fiercest but most trusted critic of his graphic design work and, as he would add, "everything else, too." Stella, clear about where she stands, says, "Even when I hate his guts I've never been bored. The day I'm bored I'm out of here." In the thirty-one years they've been together they've raised four children, renovated two houses, suffered the loss of all four of their parents, survived Stella's breast cancer, and toasted the birth of their first grandchild. This is the bright side of their story.

But in the middle of this pastoral landscape is the minefield of sex, where their worst arguments occur. She wants it; he doesn't. She wants to talk about it; he doesn't. She gets angry. He gets defensive. They clash, then wait for the dust to settle. This situation is chronic and relentless, and recently it got a lot worse.

For years, Stella has resented being the custodian of their sex life. "I'm the one who thinks about it, who wants it, who makes it happen, and who complains when it doesn't. If I left it up to James, our erotic life would be a desert." Privately James admits that he initiates only when he's reasonably sure she won't be receptive; that way, he appears to keep up his end of the bargain. Stella hates being the one who "does it all," but she doesn't dare stop, for fear that there will be nothing, an unbearable void. Better to assume his lack of interest than to confirm it.

Since Stella entered menopause her sex drive has plummeted, and her worst fears have, in fact, been confirmed. James's lack of sexual initiative, once cloaked by her eagerness, is now glaring. She feels frantic at the prospect of sexual deadness that looms before her. "We're like roommates. This time I really need him to make the effort, and he won't." I point out to Stella that even though it may look as if he won't, what's more likely is that he doesn't know how. The disruption brought about by menopause challenges a pattern that has been fixed since early in their relationship. They will soon discover that it also opens up new possibilities.

James is quick to focus on performance issues to justify his lack of desire. He foresees sexual failure, and his anxiety makes this prophecy self-fulfilling. He feels diminished and unmanly each time he fails, and his fear of impotence makes him want to stop even before he starts. The unintended irony in all this is that James becomes so obsessed with doing it right, staying hard for Stella, that he loses sight of her entirely. So while he thinks he's focusing completely on her, she feels as if he's somewhere else altogether. This has been a point of contention between them. I remark to James that holding the lens squarely on the physical act of sex—sex as a performance—is a decidedly unerotic approach. It is too narrow an angle. To me, it seems that James is overwhelmed by the whole prospect of being sexual with his wife: claiming desire, eroticizing her, feeling free to express the bawdiness of his lust with her.

When I ask James if he ever experiences anxiety-free sex, he answers, "Only when I masturbate." This is important, since it confirms for me that he has no organic difficulty and that, genitally speaking, he can perform just fine. In solitary sex James can attend to himself without the pressure of another's demands. The women who populate his fantasy life are lascivious, sexually alluring, and in no way vulnerable. He need not fear that his selfishness might hurt them, and he can delight in his excitement guilt-free. This is a freedom he never reaches with his wife, and that realization leads us to the cause of his erotic block.

James doesn't know how to enjoy himself sexually in the presence of the woman he loves. Unable to reconcile pleasing himself and pleasing Stella at the same time, he ends up pleasing neither. Even though emotionally and intellectually he is able to maintain a strong sense of himself with his wife—he hates her taste in music, refuses to wear Italian suits, and defied her by voting Republican one year—this self-possession breaks down in the sexual encounter. He fears that if he surrenders to his own concupiscence and forgets Stella, even for a moment, she will be unforgivably hurt.

Though James is not aware of this, his erotic blueprint is riddled with marks left by his relationship with his unhappy mother. When it comes to sex with Stella, he is right back to the setup he had in his childhood: he has to make an impossible choice between attending to himself and securing closeness. The guilt he felt as a child about being selfish has been transformed into sexual inhibition. Perhaps this is why James experiences his wife's desire as a demand rather than an invitation, it is an obligation, not a seduction. Eroticism has shifted into the realm of duty, and is weighted down with pressure, guilt, and worry—all proven antiaphrodisiacs.

Rekindling Desire

James and Stella are stumped. Their sex problem has been chalked up to lousy chemistry, and they think it is as permanent and irreversible as an amputated leg. For years James has been stuck in a narrative of helplessness that goes something like this: "Our problem has to be coming from somewhere; it has to be somebody's fault, and if it's not my fault, then whose fault is it? Must be Stella's. Let's blame her." Reinterpreting James's lack of desire, I locate it firmly in the reverberations of his childhood. He begins to have some compassion for himself. At the same time, I challenge him to take responsibility for it in the present. Together, we disentangle self-blame and responsibility, and map out courses of action. This brings him big relief. For Stella, this new line of attribution is a small step toward restoring her sense of self-esteem.

I work with James to establish a comfortable sense of sexual separateness, making sure to clarify that separateness does not mean indifference. Instead of fixating constantly on Stella, I ask him to do the unthinkable and hold on to himself. With this in mind, I suggest a few things. "First, leave the bedroom. Too many bad associations. Curse the bed—it has failure written all over it. It operates as a sensory deprivation tank. Find other surfaces in the house. Then, I'd like you to masturbate next to Stella, to experience the possibility of pleasing yourself in her presence. Take note of the tension and the guilt. Be mindful of them, rather than trying to avoid them."

I chose masturbation for several reasons. First, it is the one area of James's sexuality where he can let go freely. Second, it invites him to be totally self-centered, and relieves him of the responsibility of pleasing his wife. Third, it will—I hope—confirm for him that attending to himself doesn't have to hurt her. Being watched will support his ability to indulge his erotic individuality guilt-free. Finally, it will turn his performance anxiety on its head. The act of masturbating in her presence is itself a grand performance, with Stella as the sole spectator. For the first time he can consider that she may actually enjoy taking in his enjoyment. Letting her watch him roam freely in his own erotic territory is itself an intimate gift.

Each of these layers helps to create a reality that is entirely different from the one he felt with his mother. After all, we don't masturbate in front of our parents, but we can with our lovers.

Of course, when I made this suggestion I considered Stella's plight as well. When James touches her tentatively, waiting for her to give him the go-ahead, she is filled with resentment. As it turns out, James's cautious regard is a turn-off. His deference leaves her feeling burdened; his dogged focus leaves her aching. Earlier in our conversation, James made a point of telling me that Stella had a temper. "While that may be so," I confirmed, "if you had made love to her more often you would have a wife with a very different temper, because the frustration that people can experience when the body is not touched, stroked, held, and pleasured drives people up a wall. What you then get is arousal transformed into rage."

I tell Stella what I've told many people who are cherished spouses but famished lovers: "You know he loves you; you've never doubted that; and that's why you've stayed all these years. What hurts so much is that you've never felt wanted by him. You feel that it's all on you to make it happen, and indeed it is. You've forfeited sensual complicity for emotional security. It's a cruel bargain." Like a glacier suddenly melting, tears roll down Stella's face. They speak volumes about the longing and rejection she's lived with for so long. It's virtually impossible not to take such repeated denial personally, to see it as proof that one is undesirable, and to slip into self-doubt.

To James I say, "Love and desire are not the same. Cozy is not the same as sexy. Your wife knows you love her. What she wants is to feel desired by you. She wants to know your hunger, to taste the delicate flavors of your craving, and to see it as a match for her own. Your inability to let go, to surrender to your own hedonistic designs, is infuriating to her. Your passivity is irritating, and your considerateness is the opposite of her fantasy of unrestrained rapture. Your lustiness would be an open endorsement for her own ardor. It's hard to let go with someone who doesn't."

The masturbation experiment was only a partial success—it went so-so, as these things sometimes do, but there was no dramatic transformation. James's self-consciousness got the better of him. He had always marshaled masturbation as a private pleasure, and he had no desire to share it. But what happened a few days later was a real turning point. James and Stella had a row. She was upset, convinced that things would never change. His first impulse was to hold her, but he was afraid it wasn't what she wanted. She seemed so angry with him. But he pushed through his awkwardness and held her anyway. Though she wasn't responsive at first, he maintained his embrace. In the past, James had always retreated, focusing solely on her cues for readiness. He was organized by her. This time, he made his own choice, laid claim to his own feelings, and was surprisingly aroused. He rubbed her back, and she began to calm down. She knew he was there, and that he could contain her. He could withstand her intensity. One intensity dominoed another, and this led to what they both recounted separately as "wonderful lovemaking." Theirs wasn't an ecstatic fulfillment; rather, they reveled in a quiet passion, the simple understanding of two bodies reunited after a long absence.

It takes two people to create a pattern, but only one to change it. James gleefully described himself in a later session as "bold and persistent," and was amazed by how the feeling of being in charge literally charged him up. By taking control he was finally able to lose control. The sexual prison he and Stella had carefully constructed had begun to unlock. Freeing himself from his chronic reactive stance, even momentarily, filled him with hope and gave him a glimpse into the erotic possibilities that lay ahead. For the first time in years he found himself fantasizing about his wife—what they might do together, where they might do it. He reclaimed a part of himself that had been completely lost in anxiety.

It's worth pointing out that in this encounter (and subsequent ones) James had no problem with coming too soon, or even with worrying that he might. When sex feels like an obligation it's very efficacious to come fast—it brings a quick end to the discomfort. When lovers engage sexually as free agents, turning surrender into an act of self-assertion, there is no need to get it over with. Precipitating the grand finale isn't so much the point as savoring the mutual trust and intimacy along the way.

Premature ejaculation is a misnomer. It is not a matter of timing; it has to do with lack of intent. It would be better described as "involuntary ejaculation." Once James was in charge of his desire, he was in charge of his ejaculation as well.

In an interesting twist to the saga, James also told me that each time he and Stella have made love since beginning therapy it has been after an argument. "I'm a little bothered by that," he confessed. "I'd like for us to be able to make love without preceding it with whatever that is."

"Anger and excitement have a complicated relationship," I explain. "Physiologically, anger and arousal have a lot in common. Psychologically, too. In your case, I think the anger emboldens you. It relieves you of compliance, and leaves you feeling more entitled. Anger highlights separateness and is a counterpoint to dependence; this is why it can so powerfully stoke desire. It gives you the distance you need. As a habit it can be problematic, but there's no denying that it's a powerful stimulant."

Over the years I've met more than a few people like James and Stella, couples whose otherwise colorful relationship teeters on the brink of sensual austerity. Together we investigate the emotional undercurrents of their erotic stagnation. We trace the origins of the blocks as well as the relational dynamics that keep them in place. They find it useful to begin this way, and are comforted to learn that understanding the past can help them change the present.

On the Importance of Being Ruthless

We commonly believe that the closer we feel to someone, the easier it will be to shed our inhibitions. But that's only half the story. Intimacy does nurture desire, but sexual pleasure also demands separateness. Erotic excitement requires that we be able to step out of the intimate bond for a moment, turn toward ourselves, and focus on our own mounting sensations. We need to be able to be momentarily selfish in order to be erotically connected.

Our ability to step away from our loved ones while trusting their steadfastness is forged in the security of our childhood bonds.

The more we trust, the farther we are able to venture. When infants play peek a boo, the distance they can bear is only as far as the breadth of their fingers. What powers the game is the realization that, even when I don't see you, you continue to exist. Older children play hide-and-seek, secure in the knowledge that someone will eventually come looking. The thrill of hiding is followed by the relief of being found. Erotic intimacy is an adult version of hide-and-seek. As when we were children, the stronger the connection the braver we are about stretching it. We know our beloved will be waiting for our return, will not punish our selfish pursuits, and in fact may even applaud them.

In his book *Arousal*, Michael Bader links the idea of selfishness to the concept of sexual ruthlessness, which he defines as "the quality of desire that enables a person to surrender to the full force of his or her own rhythms of pleasure and excitement without guilt, worry, or shame of any kind." Bader's explanation emphasizes the importance of differentiation—the capacity to hold on to oneself in the presence of another. Without that ability, we become like James, who can't get out of Stella's head long enough to experience his own fervor.

The rawness of our desire can feel mean, bestial, even unloving. Eros can feel predatory, a voracious grab. Whatever guilt we feel about taking—whatever shame we feel about our wantonness, our passion, our indecency—is intensified in the primitive vulnerability of sex. We bring to our intimate erotic encounters a lifetime of injunctions against selfishness in the context of love, the specifics of which are detailed in our erotic blueprint. In addition to the family legacy, we also carry a cultural legacy. We are socialized to control ourselves, to restrain our impulses, to tame the animal within. So as dutiful citizens and spouses we edit ourselves and mask our ravenous appetites and conceal our fleeting need to objectify the one we love.

For many people, the prohibitions against ruthlessness within the context of a loving relationship are just too great to allow for erotic abandon. The self-absorption inherent in sexual excitement obliterates the other in a way that collides with the ideal of intimacy. Such people find they can be safely lustful and intemperate only with people they don't know as well, or care about as much. Recreational sex, pornography, and cybersex all share an element of distance, even anonymity, that avoids the burden of intimacy and makes sexual excitement possible. Clearly, these emotionally disengaged situations are more often found outside the home, where the need for differentiation is less intense. Being with an unavailable partner provides a protective limit—if you can't get too close to a person, you need not fear entrapment or loss of self.

To my thinking, cultivating a sense of ruthlessness in our intimate relationships is an intriguing solution to the problems of desire. While it may appear at first glance to be detached and even uncaring, it is in fact rooted in the love and security of our connection. It is a rare experience of trust to be able to let go completely without guilt or fretfulness, knowing that our relationship is vast enough to withstand the whole of us. We reach a unique intimacy in the erotic encounter. It transcends the civility of the emotional connection and accommodates our unruly impulses and primal appetites. The flint of rubbing bodies gives off a heat not easily achieved through tamer expressions of love. Paradoxically, ruthlessness is a way to achieve closeness. Erotic intimacy invites us into a state of unboundedness where we experience a sweet freedom. We get a temporary break from ourselves—the legacies of our childhood, the habits of our relationship, and the constraints of our respective cultures.

Loving another without losing ourselves is the central dilemma of intimacy. Our ability to negotiate the dual needs for connection and autonomy stems from what we learned as children, and often takes a lifetime of practice. It affects not only how we love but also how we make love. Erotic intimacy holds the double promise of finding oneself and losing oneself. It is an experience of merging and of total self-absorption, of mutuality and selfishness. To be inside another and inside ourselves at the same time is a double stance that borders on the mystical. The momentary oneness we feel with our beloved grows out of our ability to acknowledge our indissoluble separateness. In order to be one, you must first be two.

8

Parenthood

When Three Threatens Two

> If someone is counting on children to bring them peace of mind, self-confidence, or a steady sense of happiness, they are in for a bad shock. What children do is complicate, implicate, give plot lines to the story, color to the picture, darken everything, bring fear as never before, suggest the holy, explain the ferocity of the human mind, undo or redo some of the past while casting shadows into the future. There is no boredom with children in the home. The risks are high. The voltage crackling.
>
> —*Anne Roiphe,* Married

SEX MAKES BABIES. SO IT is ironic that the child, the embodiment of the couple's love, so often threatens the very romance that brought that child into being. Sex, which set the entire enterprise in motion, is often abandoned once children enter the picture. Even when children come by a different route, their impact on the sex life of the couple is no less dramatic. Many of the couples I see trace the demise of their erotic life back to the arrival of the first child. Why does parenthood so often deliver a fatal blow?

The transition from two to three is one of the most profound challenges a couple will ever face. It takes time—time measured in years, not weeks—to find our bearings in this brave new world.

Having a baby is a psychological revolution that changes our relation to almost everything and everyone, from our sense of self and identity to our relations with our partners, friends, parents, and in-laws. Our bodies change. So do our finances and work lives. Priorities shift, roles are redefined, and the balance between freedom and responsibility undergoes a massive overhaul. We literally fall in love with our babies and, as we once understood with our mates, falling in love is an all-consuming affair that pushes everything else aside. The making of a family calls for a redistribution of resources and, for a while, there seems to be less for the couple: less time, less communication, less sleep, less money, less freedom, less touch, less intimacy, less privacy. Even though couples talk about how happy they are as a growing family and how fulfilled they are individually, they nevertheless describe these shifts as taxing to their relationship.

Eventually, most of us come to recognize ourselves again within this new context of family. At best, we become more adept at the basic skills of caretaking. We establish the support we need. We lay out a division of labor, both domestically and professionally, that everyone can live with. We arrange for child care; we bond with other parents; we steal time in bits and pieces and get brief intermissions for ourselves. With any luck, we sleep through the night. We start going to the gym again, we finish a magazine before the next issue arrives in the mail, and we manage to create some space where we can connect with each other as adults.

For some of us, this is when romance starts to work its way back into the fabric of our lives. We remember that sex is fun; it makes us feel good, and it makes us feel closer. As my friend Clara said, "It's easy to forget that before we were parents, we were lovers. Sex reaffirms that for us. It reminds me that I chose Meyer because I love him; I'd choose him again today. For me, that's romantic."

But while some couples gravitate toward one another again, others slowly wander off on a path of mutual estrangement. Reclaiming erotic intimacy is not always easy. The case is often made that American parents today, regardless of class, are overworked and overwhelmed. As a consequence, we virtually schedule sex out of our lives, keeping it on permanent standby while we attend to more pressing matters. Family life can feel like ongoing triage: what needs my immediate attention, and what can I put off until later? We constantly sort conflicting demands into their appropriate hierarchical slots: The Crucial, The Important, The Dreamed of, The Ought-to, The Negligible, The Irrelevant, The Whatever, The Trifling, The "Maybe Someday," The "Not in this lifetime." Sex often remains firmly at the bottom of the to-do list, never relinquishing its last-place status to other, more mundane tasks.

But why does our erotic connection with our partner wind up so demoted? Does it really matter if the dishes aren't done, or is there something more beneath our mysterious willingness to forgo sex? Perhaps there is something specific about our modern American culture that reinforces the erotic muting of moms and dads. Or perhaps eroticism in the context of family is simply too difficult for anyone to embrace.

Parenthood, Inc.

Safety and stability take on a whole new meaning when children enter the picture. Read any parenting book about infants and toddlers and what you'll find over and over is an emphasis on routine, predictability, and regularity. For children to feel confident enough to go out into the world and explore on their own, they need a secure base. Parenthood demands that we become steady, dependable, and responsible. We plant ourselves firmly on the ground so that our kids may learn to fly. Even before a child arrives, we review our life insurance policies, buy a car with air bags, and move into the best (i.e., safest) neighborhood we can afford. We cut down on our drinking, finally quit smoking, and begin to keep something in the refrigerator besides a six-pack and condiments.

We do all this for our kids, but we also do it for ourselves. Facing the great unknown of parenthood, we try to establish as much security as we can. We seek to contain the unpredictable by creating structure. We organize; we prioritize; we become serious. In the process we cast aside what is frivolous, immature, irresponsible, reckless, excessive, and unproductive, for such things clash with the task at hand: building a family. "I got rid of my motorcycle when Jimmy was born. I'm not allowed to die in a bike crash anymore." "I'm a sculptor, but I took this job doing Power Point presentations for a high-end investment firm because the pay and the benefits are great and I'll be vested after five years so I won't have to worry about retirement and I can put all my extra money into Becky's college fund" (all said without the speaker taking a breath). "No partying till five o'clock in the morning for me anymore, not when I have to get up at five-thirty—six-fifteen when the baby's feeling generous." "It was all spur-of-the-moment for us before the kids. We'd decide to go camping and we'd throw the tent into the car and go. I could call Dawn at the office at five-fifteen to tell her about a band that was playing at nine, and she'd always meet me there. Now we buy season tickets but wind up giving half of them away."

Family life flourishes in an atmosphere of comfort and consistency. Yet eroticism resides in unpredictability, spontaneity, and risk. Eros is a force that doesn't like to be constrained. When it settles into repetition, habit, or rules, it touches its death. It then is transformed into boredom and sometimes, more powerfully, into repulsion. Sex, a harbinger of loss of control, is fraught with uncertainty and vulnerability. But when kids come on the scene, our tolerance for these destabilizing emotions takes a dive. Perhaps this is why they are so often relegated to the fringes of family life. What eroticism thrives on, family life defends against.

Many of us become so immersed in our role as parents that we become unable to break free, even when we might. "I knew we were in trouble when I couldn't even think about having sex until all the toys were put away," my patient Stephanie reluctantly admits. "And then there are the dishes, the laundry, the bills, the dog. The list never ends. The chores always seem to win out, and intimacy between Warren and me gets lost in the shuffle. If someone were to ask me, 'What would you rather do, mop the kitchen floor or make love to your husband?' of course I would pick sex. But in real life? I push Warren away and grab that mop."

It's easy to disparage the mop. Like a lot of mothers (yes, mothers), Stephanie resents cleaning, even while she feels compelled to pursue the tidy household as a symbol of successful motherhood. She finds herself irresistibly drawn to cleanliness, as if order on the outside can bring peace on the inside. And, to some extent, it does. As odious as her to-do list might be, there is something about getting things done that gives her a sense of control and efficacy. Enough Cheerios and Goldfish for three weeks of snack-time. Clean closets. Shoes in the next two sizes up. These are activities with immediate and measurable results, far more manageable than the open-endedness and terrors of child rearing.

Children are a blessing, a delight, a wonder. They're also a minor cataclysm. These cherished intruders fill us with a profound sense of vulnerability and lack of control. We dread the thought of something terrible happening to them or worse yet, of losing them. They hold us hostage to constant anxiety. We love them so much, and we want to protect them at all costs. We can numb these frightening thoughts or obsess about them, but in either case we want to get it right. Are they OK? How can you tell? Did I handle this well, or should we start saving up for therapy as well as college? In the face of these daunting questions, Stephanie runs for the mop, even when she doesn't have to, because it provides a modicum of control in an otherwise emotionally chaotic environment.

Actually, Stephanie used to be quite a slob. "Before I had a child I never found myself cleaning the egg cups in the refrigerator. I was messy. Books everywhere, papers everywhere, and I never experienced it as a lack of control. It felt cozy to me. But now I feel this need to exert myself over my environment. It's me against the mess, my personal battle against the forces of chaos that I know will take over the minute I turn my back to watch TV or, God forbid, to be intimate with my husband."

Before Jake was born, Stephanie worked as an office manager in an international shipping firm. She had always planned on returning to work after her maternity leave, but Jake's birth changed that. She couldn't bear the thought of leaving him; and, after doing the math, she realized that most of her paycheck would go to the babysitter anyway. Five years have passed, and Sophia has come along. "With a five-year-old and a two-year-old, I'm on mother duty twenty-four-seven. If I have any time left, I just want it for myself. When Warren approaches me, it feels like one more person wanting something from me. I know that's not his intention, but it's how I feel. I don't have anything left to give."

"When did sexual intimacy become his need only? Don't you miss the connection, too?" I ask her.

She shrugs. "Not really. I keep thinking that it will come back, but I can't say I miss it."

While Stephanie's desire has remained stagnant, Warren's frustration has risen. "I've tried everything," he tells me. "She asks for help; I give her help. I do the dishes; I let her sleep late on the weekends; I take the kids out so she can have some time to herself. But, you know, I work, too. I'm meeting deadlines all day long. It's not like I'm having a picnic. She thinks all I want is to get laid, but that's not it. I want to come home and be with my wife sometimes. But all I get is a woman who's become all mother. It's all about the kids. What we need to plan, what we need to do, what we need to buy. Can't we just give it a rest once in a while?"

"Have you seen the movie *Before Sunset*?" I ask him. "At one point the main character, Jesse, says that he feels as though he's running a day care center with someone he used to date."

"Exactly!" Warren snaps.

"Do you ever have fun?" I ask.

"Oh, we have a good time. We do a lot together as a family, and I love that. We went apple picking last weekend. We ride our bikes, go to the park, that kind of thing. The kids are fantastic; we laugh a lot. Stephanie is a terrific mom. She's always looking for something new to do together."

"Together à deux, or together with all of you?"

"Together with all of us," he grumbles.

Eros Redirected

Stephanie bursts with creativity: art projects, nature walks, trips to museums and fire stations, puppet shows, cookie cutting, cookie baking, cookie parties. Hardly a day goes by when she's not thinking about something fun and new to do with the kids. Parental love throbs with vitality. Seeing Stephanie interact with her family, it is apparent that her playful energy did not disappear when she became a mother. Her life is filled with novelty and adventure, but it all takes place in relation to her kids, leaving Warren longing. The children are the adventure now.

If we think of eroticism not as sex per se, but as a vibrant, creative energy, it's easy to see that Stephanie's erotic pulse is alive and well. But her eroticism no longer revolves around her husband. Instead, it's been channeled to her children. There are regular playdates for Jake but only three dates a year for Stephanie and Warren: two birthdays, hers and his, and one anniversary. There is the latest in kids' fashion for Sophia, but only college sweats for Stephanie. They rent twenty G-rated movies for every R-rated movie. There are languorous hugs for the kids while the grown-ups must survive on a diet of quick pecks.

This brings me to another point. Stephanie gets tremendous physical pleasure from her children. Let me be perfectly clear here: she knows the difference between adult sexuality and the sensuousness of caring for small children. She, like most mothers, would never dream of seeking sexual gratification from her children. But, in a sense, a certain replacement has occurred. The sensuality that women experience with their children is, in some ways, much more in keeping with female sexuality in general. For women, much more than for men, sexuality exists along what the Italian historian Francesco Alberoni calls a "principle of continuity." Female eroticism is diffuse, not localized in the genitals but distributed throughout the body, mind, and senses. It is tactile and auditory, linked to smell, skin, and contact; arousal is often more subjective than physical, and desire arises on a lattice of emotion.

In the physicality between mother and child lie a multitude of sensuous experiences. We caress their silky skin, we kiss, we cradle, we rock. We nibble their toes, they touch our faces, we lick their fingers, let them bite us when they're teething. We are captivated by them and can stare at them for hours. When they devour us with those big eyes, we are besotted, and so are they. This blissful fusion bears a striking resemblance to the physical connection between lovers. In fact, when Stephanie describes the early rapture of her relationship with Warren—lingering gazes, weekends in bed, baby talk, toe-nibbling—the echoes are unmistakable. When she says, "At the end of the day, I have nothing left to give," I believe her. But I also have come to believe that at the end of the day, there may be nothing more she needs.

All this play activity and intimate involvement with her children's development, all this fleshy connection, has captured Stephanie's erotic potency to the detriment of the couple's intimacy and sexuality. This is eros redirected. Her sublimated energy is displaced onto the children, who become the centerpiece of her emotional gratification.

The Cult Status of Children

The sensuous pleasure of caring for small children is natural and universal. It is also wise from an evolutionary standpoint—the mother's bond to her child is a powerful physiological response that ensures the infant's survival. However, I'd like to make a distinction between the parent-child bond, on the one hand, and a recent culture of child rearing that has inflated this bond to astonishing levels, on the other.

Stephanie's intense focus on her kids is not a mere idiosyncrasy—not simply her own personal style. In fact, this kind of overzealous parenting is a fairly recent trend that has, one hopes, reached its apex of folly. Childhood is indeed a pivotal stage of life that will inevitably shape the child's future. But the last few decades have ushered in an emphasis on children's happiness that would make our grandparents shudder. Childhood has been sanctified so that it no longer seems ridiculous for one adult to sacrifice herself entirely in order to foster the flawless and painless development of her offspring—a one-person, round-the-clock child rearing factory. This is a far cry from the days (not so long ago in America and still present in many parts of the world) when children were considered principally as collective economic assets, and women gave birth to many children in hope of keeping just a few. We no longer get work out of our children; today we get meaning.

Meanwhile, American individualism, with its emphasis on autonomy and personal responsibility, has left us between a rock and a hard place with regard to family life. On one hand, we vest our children with sentimental idealization, and we have a culture of child rearing that demands considerable emotional and material resources. On the other hand, our society notably lacks the public support necessary to complete this fundamental project. The basic services for our children—medicine, day care, and education—are beyond the reach of even many middle-class families. In our individualistic culture, we tend to "privatize" shortcomings of public policy by seeing them as personal failures. We are left with isolated domestic units: overworked parents deprived of extended families, kinship networks, and real institutional assistance. With grandma 3,000 miles away, and high-quality child care costing as much as $30,000 a year in some places (and the cost is still rising), couples are left gasping for air, space, time, and money.

The magnitude of child rearing, coupled with the scarcity of resources, affects mothers in particular, who carry most of the burden in heterosexual couples. And the problem doesn't end there; for this unprecedented child-centrality is unfolding against the backdrop of romanticism that underscores modern marraige. Not only do we want to be perfect parents and give our children everything; we also want our marital relationships to be happy, fulfilled, sexually exciting, and emotionally intimate. Indeed, in our culture the survival of the family depends on the happiness of the couple. But cultivating the ideal relationship requires care and attention, and this competes directly with the "full-contact" parenting many of us embrace. Utopian romance gets blasted by the realities of family life. Stephanie feels overwhelmed because, indeed, she is.

Warren Wants His Wife Back

Stephanie and Warren embody a common marital configuration: she is wrapped up in the kids, exhausted, and uninterested in sex; he is frustrated and lonely. She resents the fact that everything having to do with the kids and the house falls squarely on her shoulders, and she claims that if he were more helpful she'd be more inclined toward sex. She wishes they could sometimes be physical without having to go straight to sex, and complains that his demands are proof of his insensitivity. She alternates between resentment and guilt.

Warren feels displaced, and claims that he's been fed a litany of excuses for years. "First she was too nauseated, then she was too tired, then she was too big. After Jake was born, it was the episiotomy, the nursing, the sore nipples. 'Not now, I'm nursing Jake. Not now, I just finished nursing Jake. Not now, I have to nurse Jake later.' Then she was too fat, too out of shape. We got it together briefly when we were trying to conceive Sophia, but now we're right back to zero." By the time they come to see me, they're locked in a pattern. He initiates; she rebuffs him; he feels rejected and withdraws; she feels emotionally bereft and even more distrustful of his sexual motives. "We don't get along well enough for me to even try," she complains. They blame one another for their sexual unhappiness, and each holds the other responsible for making it better.

I am worried about them, and I let them know it. This is not because I think that a couple can't have a viable relationship without sex—the absence of sexual desire, when it is mutual, is not necessarily an indicator of dissatisfaction. There are a lot of ways to be happily committed, and not all of them include sex. However, if one partner really misses sex and can't engage the other, a pernicious downward spiral is set in motion. For these chronically disappointed partners, the absence of sexual intimacy creates an emotional desert. Sooner or later things come to a head. They rebel and find sex elsewhere: on line, or in flings, tricks, or affairs. Or they leave, even if that means waiting till the kids grow up. Or they stay but grow so bitter and resentful that you wish they'd leave. Warren and Stephanie seem headed in a troubling direction.

What Stephanie fails to see is that behind Warren's nagging insistence is a yearning to be intimate with his wife. For him, sex is a prelude to intimacy, a pathway to emotional vulnerability. She responds to him as if he were one more needy child. She doesn't realize that this is not just for him but for her, too. Like a lot of women, once she's in the caretaking mode she has a hard time switching it off. She's so mentally organized in terms of what she does for everyone else that she is unable to recognize when something is offered to her.

What Warren finds intolerable is that his approach is having the opposite effect of what he intends. He is desperate for a flicker of desire from Stephanie, but he wants it just to be there, sudden and whole, the way it is for him. I explain to him that expecting our partner to be in the mood just because we are is a setup for disappointment. We take lack of desire as a personal rejection, and forget that one of the great elixirs of passion is anticipation. You can't force desire, but you can create an atmosphere where desire might unfurl. You can listen, invite, tease, kiss. You can tempt, compliment, romance, and seduce. All these tactics help to compose an erotic substratum from which your partner can more easily be lifted.

Even before Stephanie had children, her sexuality was always more receptive than initiating, and she rarely experienced spontaneous desire. In those days, Warren's role was lavishly complementary: her coyness was dissipated by his assertiveness. He not only made her feel desired and desirable; he also made her feel desirous. He would entice her slowly, gradually awakening her senses, and she would eagerly respond. This responsiveness, so marked in the early days of their courtship, temporarily masked her characteristic lack of sexual agency (a trait shared by many women).

I point out to him that she might be more receptive today if he paid attention to cultivating her desire rather than simply monitoring it. For Stephanie, love and desire are inseparable. She needs to feel intimate before she can allow the vulnerability of sex; otherwise, she feels objectified. "Sometimes it feels like he just wants a release. It has nothing to do with me," she says. "It's a total turn-off."

"Stephanie needs you to take the lead, but you can't just buy her a ticket; you have to get her interested in the trip," I tell Warren. "You play an important role as the keeper of the flame. Right now, all she feels is pressure. She experiences your come-ons as abrupt and intrusive. She thinks all you want is sex. Prove to her it's not."

Looking for Stephanie

It was harder for me to reach Stephanie, for she and I could not easily separate ourselves from the ideological pressures that lurked beneath the surface of our conversation. Validating her husband's needs could easily be construed as denying hers. How to invite a woman to reconnect with her body and her sexuality, separately from her children, when she's completely uninterested in either, or when she feels undeserving or too maxed out? How to avoid the pitfall of swinging back and forth between her children's needs and her husband's needs, leaving her own needs perennially unattended? I did not want to impose a bias about sex that would add more pressure to the mix.

What I said to her was this, "You'll never hear me say that you should force yourself. Nothing is more deflating erotically than sex on demand. But I do believe that sex matters: for you, for your marriage, and for your kids. I am puzzled by your willingness to forgo such an important part of yourself. How did it come to be that, on the extensive list of things your children need, parents who have sex isn't one of them?"

Many women struggle to integrate sexuality and motherhood. Ours is a culture that equates maternal devotion with selflessness: self-sacrifice, self-abnegation, self-denial. Stephanie has had years of putting the children first and forgetting herself altogether. She has relinquished her freedom and her independence—both cornerstones of desire—and has forsaken herself as a person in her own right. Reconnecting with her erotic self, separate from her maternal self, is crucial. Together we probe the elusiveness of her sexual agency. We explore her sexual history: how sexuality was expressed in her family while she was growing up, and what her earliest experiences were like. She tells me how awkward her own mother was about the subject of sex, never speaking frankly but only making veiled references to morality and sin. She has never thought of her mother as a sexual being, and it doesn't escape me that history might be repeating itself.

We talk about how her sexual identity changed as a result of pregnancy, childbirth, nursing, and motherhood. Putting her personal experiences in a broader cultural context, we discuss how the politics of motherhood, the myth of chastity, and the medicalization of pregnancy and childbirth all conspire to deprive motherhood of its sexual elements. I recommend a gem of a book: *Sexy Mamas*, by Cathy Winks and Anne Semans, which discusses sexuality and motherhood in an accessible, down-to-earth, positive way. I suggest she leave it in plain view on her bedside table.

These conversations were an attempt to reintroduce sex to Stephanie's psychic landscape, and help her to get a sense of herself as a sexual being. For years, she has consigned her desire to Warren, who has been slated for their erotic upkeep (along with the snow tires, the lawn, and the garbage). I know we are on to something when she blurts out, "I've been a sexual underachiever my whole life, and I resent Warren for feeling entitled to something that I won't allow for myself!"

Together we shift the focus from self-denial to self-awareness. We explore how she might reclaim a right to pleasure, with its inherent threat of selfishness, in a way that doesn't leave her feeling like a bad mother. One upshot of these discussions is that Stephanie does something radical (for her)—she goes on a weekend retreat with her sister, leaving Warren and the children to their own devices. Getting to that point took a lot of work, but I sense that before she can open herself to sex, she needs to expand the general domain of personal pleasure. Becoming more generous with herself, she might—I hope—be more receptive to her husband.

I'm not big on homework in therapy, especially when the list of domestic tasks is already endless. At the same time, action is a prerequisite for change. So I ask Warren and Stephanie, at the end of one session, to each do one thing differently in the next few weeks. They need not talk about it, for their effort will be measured not by its success but only by its intention. "I'd like you to stretch, to do something, anything, that takes you a step farther than usual." To Warren I say, "We tend to do for others what we would like them to do for us, but it isn't necessarily what they might want. Part of this is about working with and honoring your differences. At one time you pursued Stephanie with great creativity, but no more. There's an assumption—and you're not alone—that we need only pursue what we don't yet possess. The trick is that in order to keep our partner erotically engaged we have to become more seductive, not less."

At this point, sex has been relegated to what Warren wants and what Warren misses. Stephanie has shifted from being receptive to being reactive. It is a passive stance in which her main power is that of refusal. To her I suggest, "Keep in mind that there's something limiting about an absolute no. What really hurts him is categorical rejection. You might find more freedom in 'Maybe' or 'Let's kiss' or even 'Talk me into it.' Warren, more than anyone else, can help you to reconnect with the woman inside the mother. Can you imagine recruiting him rather than pushing him away? Invite him to invite you, and see what happens."

Stephanie, consumed by motherhood, was too quick to dismiss the inherent value of Warren's persistence. The way I see it, Warren provides a consistent reminder that erotic intimacy matters. With him, and through him, she potentially can begin to disentangle from the bond with her children and transfer some of her energy back to herself and her relationship with Warren. When the father reaches out to the mother, and the mother acknowledges him, redirecting her attention, this serves to rebalance the entire family. Boundaries get drawn, and new zoning regulations get put in place delineating areas that are adult only. Time, resources, playfulness, and fun are redistributed, and libido is rescued from forced retirement.

My work with gay and lesbian couples has led me to recognize that these dynamics are replicated whenever one parent, gender notwithstanding, takes charge of the kids. Since same-sex couples are not constrained by a traditional division of labor—women at home, men at work—they offer a useful basis for comparison. What I see over and over is that the person who takes on the role of primary caretaker almost always undergoes changes similar to Stephanie's: a total immersion in the lives and rhythms of the children, a loss of self, and a greater difficulty extricating himself or herself from chores (a compulsion that is simultaneously frustrating and grounding).

The role of the more autonomous parent is to help the primary caregiver disengage from the kids and reallocate energy to the couple. "Leave the toys for now, nobody is going to give you a medal, go take a nap." "You don't have to make these pecan pies from scratch, you've done enough today." "The nanny is here, let's sit down for ten minutes and share a glass of wine before she leaves." It's a different approach from the traditional division of labor, one which emphasizes shared responsibility and mutuality and honors the interdependent agency of both partners.

When Warren asks, "Want to?" and Stephanie finally answers, "Convince me," their dynamic begins to shift. This puts a halt to the grinding antagonism and introduces an overdue mutuality. Asking him to help her is, in itself, an expression of sexual assertiveness. And Warren, finally relieved of being the supplicant, can set out to get his wife back. His role as keeper of the flame is given new meaning.

Lifting the Erotic Embargo

Warren and Stephanie are headed in the right direction, but the forces of eros are not yet aligned. Warren's most elaborate seduction rituals are thwarted, repeatedly and pitifully, by an unaccommodating home life. There is something absurd about the extent to which their lives revolve around their children: weekends filled with Pee Wee baseball and birthday parties; kids who go to bed a mere half hour before their parents; an open-door policy for the marital bed. In six years, Warren and Stephanie have not spent a single weekend together, away from their kids. They have stopped factoring their own needs into the family budget, and a babysitter is considered a rare luxury rather than a vital necessity. Simply put, they have never carved out the time and space they need to unwind and replenish themselves, either as individuals or as a couple. No longer focused on one another, they have turned to the children to compensate for what they are missing.

I have noticed over the years that child-centrality isn't just a matter of lifestyle; it is sometimes an emotional configuration as well. Children are indeed a source of nurturance for adults. Their unconditional love and utter devotion infuse our lives with a heightened sense of meaning. The problem arises when we turn to them for what we no longer get from each other: a sense that we're special, that we matter, that we're not alone. When we transfer these adult emotional needs onto our children, we are placing too big a burden on them. In order to feel safe, kids need to know that there are limits to their power, and to what is surreptitiously asked of them. They need us to have our own loving relationships, in whatever form they take. When we are emotionally and sexually satisfied (at least reasonably so; let's not get carried away here), we allow our children to experience their own independence with freedom and support.

If Warren and Stephanie are going to get their groove back, they need to free themselves, both emotionally and practically, from the disproportionate focus on their kids. Spontaneity is desirable, but the reality of family life demands planning. Couples without kids can initiate sex on a whim, but parents need to be more practical. Be it a regular date night, a weekend away every few months, or an extra half hour in the car, what matters is that couples cordon off erotic territory for themselves. When Warren and Stephanie balk at the idea of premeditated sex, I respond, "Planning can seem prosaic, but in fact it implies intentionality, and intentionality conveys value. When you plan for sex, what you're really doing is affirming your erotic bond. It's what you did when you were dating. Think of it as prolonged foreplay—from twenty minutes to two days."

Planning has proved to be most useful for Stephanie. She elaborates, "Warren's idea of a date is this: he approaches me for sex at eleven on Tuesday, and when I turn him down he says, 'Can we have a date tomorrow night?' I've had to explain to him that, for me, scheduled intercourse is not a date. I need to go out. I want food that someone else has cooked, on dishes that someone else is going to wash. When we go out, we talk, we kiss, we joke. We can finish a sentence without being interrupted. He pays attention to me, and it makes me feel sexy."

Not only do their rendezvous help maintain the emotional connection so critical for Stephanie; they also help her to make the transition from full-time mom to lover. "For so long, my thinking about sex was about how to avoid it. Knowing that Warren and I have a date has helped me to anticipate it instead. I pamper myself. I take a shower, shave my legs, put on makeup. I make a special effort to block the negativity and to give myself permission just to be sexual."

The story of Stephanie and Warren is typical of the effect of parenthood on eroticism, but it is only one among many. It is the story of a straight, white, legally married, middle-class couple whose egalitarian ideals and romantic aspirations were mercilessly undone in the transition from two to three. My work with them isn't finished. Things have definitely improved, but for this couple, and for this woman, caring for small kids doesn't agree with eroticism. I suspect that when they reach the next life stage—when the kids are both in school full time and Stephanie is back at work, as she plans—new energy will be released. In the meantime, thinking of this as but one phase in a lifelong relationship helps them remain patient and hopeful.

Sexy Mamas Do Exist

Today we arrive at parenthood with a sexual identity that's often fully sprung. All of us benefited when sexuality was cut loose from reproduction. As regular users of birth control, we have been granted the privilege of a risk-free romp that can go on for years. We enjoy desire with impunity, at least for a time, and we expect sexual fulfillment in our committed relationships. For our parents and grandparents, sex after kids probably wasn't all that different from sex before kids—pregnancy, and the heavy responsibility that went with it, was always a looming possibility. But for baby boomers and all who have followed, parenthood throws a wrench into our liberated, self-gratifying lifestyle. The "baby clash" is all the more galling because we have something to compare it with. "You used to love sex," "We used to make love for hours," and "I used to know how to turn you on," are laments I frequently hear. We're as flabbergasted as we are resentful when parenthood brings our fun to a screeching halt.

Both men and women face these changes, but not in the same way and certainly not equally. The liberation that so bolstered women's sexuality has yet to cross the threshold of motherhood, which has not lost the aura of morality and even sanctity that it always had. Desexualization of the mother is a mainstay of traditionally patriarchal cultures, which makes the sexual invisibility of modern western mothers seem particularly acute. Perhaps it's our Puritan legacy that strips motherhood of its sexual components; perhaps we are convinced that lustfulness conflicts with maternal duty.

Of course, there is more than one America, and cultural differences abound within this vast country. My friend June is quick to remind me that not all Americans came here on the *Mayflower*. "Black people are certainly not spared our share of sex problems, but we're definitely a lot less hung up than you white folks," she says. "Sex is a natural part of life, not some big dirty secret. My kids know I have sex; I knew my parents had sex. They'd put on Marvin Gaye, shut the bedroom door, and tell us we'd better not knock." My Argentinean girlfriend jokes about how her husband calls her "mamita" in bed—what better way to co-opt the taboo? My Spanish colleague Susanna tells me that, in Madrid, her greatest sexual asset is her beautiful three-year-old son. "In New York it's my accent, my hair, my legs, but definitely not my son." My American patient Stacey, a white woman who lives in Brooklyn with her daughter, knows her demographics. "The only men who flirt with me are the West Indian pediatrician, the Russian dentist, the Italian baker, and the Puerto Rican grocer. The white guys? Forget it. If I'm with my kid, they look right past me." A man with a baby in tow gets a very different response. It's not just power that is an aphrodisiac. A guy walking down the street with a toddler on his shoulders projects stability, commitment, and nurturing. For most women (and some gay men), that's sexy.

In his book *Paris to the Moon*, Adam Gopnik contrasts America's asexual model of reproduction with the more voluptuous French view, "All American What-to-Expect books begin with the Test, not the Act." He goes on, "In Paris, [pregnancy] is something that has happened because of sex, which with help and counsel, can end with your being set free to go out and have more sex. In New York, pregnancy is a ward in the house of Medicine. In Paris, it is a chapter in a sentimental education, a strange consequence of the pleasures of the body."

Despite the pervasiveness of the American mind-set, there are plenty of women who mount daily insurrections against the denial of eros. For them, motherhood heralds newfound sexual confidence, womanliness, and even the restitution of a wounded body. One day, I had back-to-back sessions, first with Stephanie, then with Amber. The realities of their daily lives had an uncanny resemblance, but their experiences couldn't have been farther apart. Amber told me, "I used to say no to sex as a matter of course. Who knows why? Denial of any desire, even hunger, was modeled for me by my 105-pound mother. Before I had kids, whenever my husband asked me if I wanted to eat, I also said no. I refused out of habit, before actually registering the question.

"Now I know far more profound reasons to say no to sex:

the desperate fatigue of new motherhood; the seemingly bottomless rage at my two-and-a-half-year-old for waking up his sleeping infant brother; the bitterness of feeling unsupported, a workhorse for our home and children. And yet I am the one who feels hungry for sex, who demands it or mopes about not getting it. I give all day in very physical ways: nursing, cooking, stooping to pick up toys, carrying children, changing diapers. After a few days of peanut butter sandwiches and Wiggles CDs, when I am a participant in my children's world to the exclusion of my own, I want my glass of sherry, my music, and my man. I long to be yanked out of the messy hair, spit-up-on shirt, mac-and-cheese-encrusted jeans that I think of as the 'mother body.' As often as I can, I put that body to bed with the kids."

Another patient, Charlene, is being tutored by her children. "My kids have taught me how to be greedy. My fifteen-month-old can suck on me for half an hour, walk off to play, and be back for more within minutes. He shakes his head no when I offer him milk in a cup or bottle, pulls up my shirt, and squeals until I unsnap my bra for him. When he sees my nipple he smiles, coos, and dives in. The three-year-old wants my lap, my time, my attention as often as he can steal it from his brother. He will tell me how to position my body on the floor, exactly how I should push the truck, and feels no guilt or shame in declaring which parent he wants to play with or put him to bed. Of course they don't always get what they want, but I am impressed by their fluid transmission of desire between body and mind. They let themselves feel in a way I'd forgotten, or been trained away from; and watching them makes me more aware of my own body and reminds me of my own desire."

For Renee, pregnancy ushered in a self-acceptance she had never felt. "Pregnancy was a healing experience for me. I was sexually abused as a child, and had always loathed any signs of womanliness in my body. I'd been at war with my thighs for twenty-five years. I was hospitalized for an eating disorder the year before I got pregnant. In fact, I was so skinny I didn't even think I could get pregnant. I hadn't had a regular period in years. But the minute I saw that plus sign in the EPT everything changed. It was the first time in my life that food became decontaminated. I relished watching my body grow ripe. For once in my life my breasts were naturally round and I was so proud. Most of my friends complained of the discomfort and weight gain. But for me, I felt like it was finally OK to look like a woman. I gave birth naturally; it was powerful. I was amazed by what my body could do and what it could endure. I was capable of so much more than I thought. Ever since, when I make love, I pursue that intensity."

For Julie, a mother of three, motherhood has brought a positive new identity. "In my early twenties I dressed like a boy: big sweaters, jeans, size-nine Keds. It was a total denial of femininity and a feminist distrust of its motives. I mistook appreciation for objectification, and didn't trust that a man might be interested in me beyond my availability as a sexual object. These days the pants are stylish, tight, and fun; the blouses show cleavage. Finally, I'm the kind of woman my Italian father would recognize, and who would make my mother blush—greedy, sexy, entitled. Why? I feel safe now. I have no one's eye to catch. I'm already caught, thoroughly enmeshed in the needs and desires of others (four males as it turns out). And I am finding freedom in this place, where there is no power game. I don't have to respond to anyone I haven't already chosen. As a mother I'm not afraid to be sexual, sensual, to assert my desire."

When Daddy Sings the Baby Blues

For every man like Warren, who feels sexually abandoned when his wife becomes a mother, there is a man like Leo, whose libido makes a break for it on the way home from the delivery room. Dwindling desire in mothers is, in some ways, old news. We might not like it, but we can at least make sense of it. But what are we to make of the father who can no longer eroticize the mother of his children? This story, though just as common, is admitted far less frequently.

When Carla and Leo came to see me, she was at her wit's end. They'd been together seventeen years: the first six a frenzy of the flesh, the next four the chaos of babyhood, the last seven a sexual desert. She went from talking to pleading to screaming to compensating. She had a number of flings and then a serious affair. He found out, she threatened divorce, he suggested therapy, and here they are.

She says, "I am so sick of the excuses. It's his work, it's the stress, it's his dying father, he has to get up early, he hasn't been to the gym and so he doesn't have the energy, his back hurts, it's my breath, it's my weight, it's his weight. I took it personally for so long, but now I'm done. I love this man, I'm prepared to stay, but I can't live like this."

He says, "I always considered myself to be very competent sexually. We kid around that we broke furniture when we first started dating; there was a lot of passion. I never looked at the kids as a defining moment in my life sexually, but obviously something switched somewhere deep inside."

I learn that Leo had begun to withdraw physically when Carla became pregnant with their first son, and they had no sexual contact at all during the last trimester. Leo just came home later and later from work. Carla knew something was up, though they never discussed it openly.

"What changed for you when she became a mother?" I ask.

"Her significance," he answers. "Her whole being turned from being my lover, my partner, and my wife to being the mother of my son. And then the mother of my other son. For a while they needed her completely, and that was really OK with me. I thought it was the most awesome thing in the world to have our babies sleeping next to us, for her to nurse them through the night. I wasn't jealous at all. I'm a very loving, nurturing father myself."

"What's it like to suck the breast of a woman who's been nursing a baby?" I ask him.

"It was weird," he answered. "The whole physical thing was a little weird. I watched her give birth, twice, and I've got to say it was not so great for our sex life."

"I know it's supposed to be this magical moment, the miracle of life and all that, but no one seems to want to acknowledge the yuck factor," I reassure him. "It's not politically correct for a man to admit that watching his wife give birth can be gross. There's a character in one of Alice Walker's books, I think it's Mr. Hal, who watches his partner give birth and is never able to touch her—or any other woman—for the rest of his life. He says he never wants to put someone through that again."

"That's a little extreme, but yeah. I became different with her, more cautious, not as free. I guess it stopped me from being aggressive or passionate or desiring her in that way—really giving myself to her, or taking her, when normally that's how we were together. It was definitely a shift."

"Couldn't do that to the mother of your children?" I ask.

"Apparently not," he answers.

"Let's talk about this whole Madonna/whore business," I continue. "It has deep psychological roots. A lot of men find it difficult to eroticize the mother of their children. It feels too regressive, too incestuous, too oedipal. What you need to remember is that she's their mom, not yours. At this point, I recommend anything that can introduce a little healthy objectification. Anything that might distinguish her from 'the mother.'"

Carla had been quiet for much of the session, but the following week I had no doubt she'd been paying attention. Laughing, she told me the story.

"I really wanted to let go with Leo. I wanted to give him an involved, prolonged, great blow job. Not just the compulsory head, not just the polite head. But I knew there was this thing with the wife, 'the mother.' Would he let me? So I initiated this game and said, 'You know, we can have a couple of different kinds of sex and you can call it what you will, but if you want this blow job to continue it's going to cost you.' I said, 'A hundred bucks if you want that kind of head. A hundred bucks.' I thought the money would be fun, but I was really into seeing if Leo could de-role that mother. Well, you don't pay the mother of your kids for a blow job, do you? You don't pay your wife for a blow job. It was a lovely experiment, that's all I'm going to say."

"Maybe you could start taking credit cards. Keep a credit card machine by the bed," Leo jokes.

Carla's playful erotic intervention has stayed with me for years. In one gesture she cleverly captured and subverted the whole issue: how to retrieve the lover from the mother. Leo feared expressing the rawness of his desire to the mother of his children, a woman too worthy of love and respect. Carla took a risk, interrupted the pattern, and invited him into an erotic complicity. She uncloaked the repression and became a sexually provocative, slutty woman who demanded to be paid. In the midst of this explicitly staged endorsement of blatant sexuality, Leo's lustfulness was finally unleashed.

Escaping the Siege of Family Life

Having a child is one of our grand aspirations. In a way we reproduce, be it biologically or through the other ways we create a family, so as not to die. We carve a place in the cycle of life and become inscribed in the course of history. We extend ourselves beyond mortality by leaving something, some one, behind: a representative of our union. In this way, having a child speaks of desire. It is a pure, life-affirming act. How cruel to see it erode the force that brought it into being.

There is no question that children make the erotic connection more difficult to sustain. There are the demands for routine without which family life cannot function, but which undermine sexual spontaneity. There is the undeniable stress on the couple's resources: less time, money, and energy to spend on each other. There is the sexual invisibility of the American mother, which is so deeply rooted in our psyche that men and women alike conspire to deny maternal sexuality. There are the many ways we shut ourselves down sexually in the family, acting under the assumption that we need to keep sex hidden from children in order to protect them.

For many parents, the idea of a secret garden inspires everything from acute guilt and anxiety to the more benign gradations of embarrassment. We are afraid that our adult sexuality will somehow damage our kids, that it's inappropriate or dangerous. But whom are we protecting? Children who see their primary caregivers at ease expressing their affection (discreetly, within appropriate boundaries) are more likely to embrace sexuality with the healthy combination of respect, responsibility, and curiosity it deserves. By censoring our sexuality, curbing our desires, or renouncing them altogether, we hand our inhibitions intact to the next generation.

There are so many reasons to give up on sex that those who don't are champions in their own right. The brave and determined couples who maintain an erotic connection are, above all, the couples who value it. When they sense that desire is in crisis, they become industrious, and make intentional, diligent attempts to resuscitate it. They know that it is not children who extinguish the flame of desire; it is adults who fail to keep the spark alive.

9

Of Flesh and Fantasy

In the Sanctuary of the Erotic Mind
We Find a Direct Route to Pleasure

The whole fauna of human fantasies, their marine vegetation, drifts and luxuriates in the dimly lit zones of human activity, as though plaiting thick tresses of darkness. Here, too, appear the lighthouses of the mind, with their outward resemblance to less pure symbols. The gateway to mystery swings open at the touch of human weakness and we have entered the realms of darkness. One false step, one slurred syllable together reveal a man's thoughts.

—*Louis Aragon*

WHEN CATHERINE HIT PUBERTY SHE was fifty pounds overweight. Sexually invisible, repeatedly rejected, she was the "ugly sidekick" left guarding the door while her girlfriends made out on the other side of it. Today she is a beautiful woman, married for almost fifteen years. She and her husband play out a fantasy in which she is a high-priced prostitute. Men pay top dollar for the pleasure of her company—they want her so much they're willing to spend a small fortune and risk their jobs and marriages for a little bit of her time. The more outrageous their transgressions, the greater her value. Catherine's past humiliations are vindicated by the men who now can't walk past her without marveling. In her theater of the surreal she triumphantly exacts revenge for the pains and frustrations of her adolescence.

Daryl's wife complains, "He can't even decide on a restaurant, and he wants to tie me up? What's that about?" The difficulty Daryl feels about asserting himself in his daily life is spectacularly remediated in his domination fantasies. In the highly ritualized and consensual choreography of bondage and domination, Daryl's aggression finds safe expression. His wants are honored, his fear of going too far is contained, and his masculine power brings others pleasure rather than pain.

Lucas, an unabashedly gay man who grew up in a small town in southern Illinois, spent years passing for straight, terrified that he'd be found out. He played high school football and even had sex with a cheerleader because she approached him in a crowd and he knew that turning her down would raise suspicions about his sexuality. Now in his thirties, he says, "I got the hell out of that town so I could be openly gay without it threatening my life. And now I find myself walking the nude beach at Aquinnah pretending to be straight so some guy can try to turn me. I'll be straight, but on my terms. Today I only act straight when I think it'll get me laid. Lucky for me, so many gay men get off on turning a straight guy that I get laid all the time!"

Emir is a one-woman man, and has been his whole life. "I've always had girlfriends, real girlfriends, women I've loved whom I've stayed with for years. That's me. I've been with Althea for five years now. We used to have a great sex life, but since we had a baby six months ago she doesn't want sex nearly as often as she used to. I have to deploy my whole seductive arsenal to convince her, and sometimes even that doesn't work. Most of the time I take care of myself." Emir's favorite fantasy is having sex with two women at once. "I like the idea of all that attention."

Many straight men fantasize variations on the theme of the

omni-sexual woman. She doesn't have to be wooed or coaxed into sex. She doesn't have to get in the mood, because she's always in the mood. She doesn't say, "How can you think about sex now when we have so much stuff to do?" She says, "More, more, more." She doesn't make him feel bad for wanting sex, because she wants it just as much. When two French maids invite you into their bed, you can be sure that neither one of them is going to say, "Not tonight, honey, I'm too tired."

Poor Man's Bread

Until recently, sexual fantasy has gotten a bad rap. What Christianity viewed as a sin later became, in the eyes of modern psychology, a perversion limited to the dissatisfied and the immature. Even today, many people believe that fantasy is nothing more than thin compensation for libidinal frustration and lack of opportunity due to failure of nerve, arrested development, or a paunch. They believe that what we fantasize about sexually is what we want to have happen in reality. "If my husband was really attracted to me he wouldn't need to look at pictures of women with big boobs," complains one wife. "When I fantasize about other men ravishing me, I feel like I'm betraying my boyfriend," says another client. "What kind of woman wants to be raped?"

I, too, used to take the narrow view that fantasy was the poor man's bread—the meal of the sensually impoverished. I had been taught to regard fantasies as a symptom of neurosis or immaturity, or as erotically tinged romantic idealizations that blind one to his or her partner's true identity and undermine real-life relationships. I was stuck at the border between the imaginary and the real, diverted from delving into the complexity of the erotic mind. Luckily, I was curious enough to ask my patients about their fantasy lives. But once they told me, I still didn't know what to do with the information. It was like watching a great Russian movie without subtitles; I had no idea what it was about, though I could appreciate the beauty of the cinematography.

Over the years, the thinking in the field has evolved, so that we now look at fantasy as a natural component of healthy adult sexuality. From an almost exclusive focus on fantasies as furtive compulsions (or perverse wishes of an unfulfilled minority), the view has widened. The collective work of philosophers and clinicians like Michel Foucault, Georges Bataille, Ethel Spector Person, Robert Stoller, Jack Morin, Michael Bader, and dozens of others has brought about a sea change in grasping the depth and richness of the erotic imagination: what it is, and what it can do.

In my own practice, I've come to view fantasy as a valuable imaginative resource, whether it is cultivated by individuals or jointly by couples. The ability to go anywhere in our imagination is a pure expression of individual freedom. It is a creative force that can help us transcend reality. By giving us an occasional escape from a relationship, it serves as a powerful antidote to loss of libido within the relationship. Simply put, love and tenderness are enriched by the spice of imagination.

Fantasies—sexual and other—also have nearly magical powers to heal and renew. They return the breasts confiscated by mastectomy, or let us walk as we did before the crippling accident. They reverse time, making us young again, and briefly allow us to be as we no longer are and maybe never were: flawless, strong, beautiful. They put us in the presence of the beloved who has died, or bring back memories of passionate lovemaking with the partner we now struggle to eroticize. Through fantasy we repair, compensate, and transform. For a few moments, we rise above the reality of life and, subsequently, the reality of death.

The more I listen and probe, the more I appreciate the shrewdness of fantasy—its energy, its imaginative efficiency, its healing qualities, and its psychological force. Our fantasies combine the uniqueness of our personal history with the broad sweep of the collective imagination. Each culture uses incentives and prohibitions to convey what is sexy (*American Idol*! Monica Lewinsky!) and what is forbidden (altar boys! Monica Lewinsky!). Our flights of fancy bridge the gap between the possible and the permissible. Fantasy is the alchemy that turns this jumble of psychic ingredients into the pure gold of erotic arousal.

In my work with couples, sexual fantasy also provides a wellspring of information about the individuals' internal life and the relational dynamics of the couple. Fantasies are an ingenious way our creative mind overcomes all sorts of conflicts around desire and intimacy. The psychoanalyst Michael Bader (whose incisive book *Arousal* discusses the undercurrents of fantasy) explains that in the sanctuary of the erotic mind, we find a psychological safe space to undo the inhibitions and fears that roil within us. Our fantasies allow us to negate and undo the limits imposed on us by our conscience, by our culture, and by our self-image.

If we feel insecure and unattractive, in our fantasies we are irresistible. If we anticipate a withholding woman, in fantasy she's insatiable. If we fear our own aggression, in our internal reveries we can feel powerful without worrying that we might hurt another. If we don't dare ask, in our erotic imaginings the other knows our needs even before we do. If we feel we shouldn't have sex, in our private theater we can surrender to a lustful other without having to bear the responsibility—we did what he wanted, it wasn't us. Fantasy expresses the problem and provides the solution. It is a fervid space, where our inhibiting fear is transformed into brazenness. What a relief to find that our shame is now curiosity, our timidity is now assertiveness, and our helplessness is now sovereignty.

Fantasy does not, however, always take the form of elaborate, scripted scenarios. Many people think that if they don't fantasize with carefully orchestrated plots and well-drawn characters, then they're not fantasizing at all. This is particularly true of women, who seem to have a harder time owning their sexual thoughts in general. My patient Claudia once described to me, in great detail, how she would like her husband to approach her. She envisioned a slow, gradually unfolding dance of seduction throughout the day, with tantalizing conversations, light kisses on the nape, gentle touches, warm smiles, and sidelong glances. "I want him to touch my arm without touching my breast. I want him to tease me, to move in a bit sexually and then pull back, to make me want. I want to *ask* him to touch my breast," she explains.

"And if he did these things?" I ask.

"We would have an entirely different sexual relationship," she answers.

Not twenty minutes later, when I ask her about her fantasy life, she assures me, "I don't fantasize. Jim does, but I don't. He's all into threesomes." I am stunned. I say, "Are you kidding? Your entire description of foreplay and anticipation is fantasy. It's certainly not reality, is it?"

To my thinking, sexual fantasy includes any mental activity that generates desire and intensifies enthusiasm. These thoughts need not be graphic, or even well-defined. They're often inarticulate, more feelings than images, more sensuous than sexual. Virtually anything can work its way into one's erotic imagination. Memories, smells, sounds, words, specific times of the day, textures—all can be considered fantasy as long as they set in motion the arc of desire.

In her book *Men in Love*, Nancy Friday writes:

> A fantasy is a map of desire, mastery, escape, and obscuration; the navigational path we invent to steer ourselves between the reefs and shoals of anxiety, guilt, and inhibition. It is a work of consciousness, but in reaction to unconscious pressures.

What is fascinating is not only how bizarre fantasies are, but how comprehensible; each one gives us a coherent and consistent picture of personality—the unconscious—of the person who invented it, even though he may think it the random whim of the moment.

Silence, Please!

The symbolic paradoxes and the irrationality of our erotic mindscape provide the most fascinating and revealing glimpse into our depths. Fantasies express truths about ourselves that are hard to get at otherwise. They reveal us at our most bare, and in their own mysterious way they convey our deepest wishes.

Yet when it comes to talking about our internal musings, most of us are remarkably tight-lipped, even with our partners (perhaps especially with our partners). In an age where intimacy is organized around disclosing uncomfortable personal truths, erotic silence holds steady as the norm. Though we may be comfortable talking about what we do, few of us are keen to reveal what we're thinking while we do it.

At the most basic level, our reluctance stems from simple embarrassment. Most of us were taught at a very young age to keep our thoughts to ourselves and our hands off our bodies. Some of us were handed down a stricter message that turned our innocent curiosity into lasting shame. Schooled in silence, the inheritors of an incontrovertible distrust of sex, it is no wonder we're filled with discomfort at the prospect of conveying our innermost thoughts. By opening ourselves to another, we risk being laughed at and judged. My patient Zoya summed it up well: "The way I grew up, there was no liking sex, let alone talking about it. People who have sex because they like it are all sluts and perverts who go blind and grow hair on their palms. You bet I kept my mouth shut."

If we're not talking, no one else is, either. Many of us experience our sexual fantasies in isolation (despite the public ubiquitousness of sex). Since we don't know what others are thinking and doing, we have nothing to compare ourselves with, no way to gauge whether or not we're normal. We're afraid of being different and therefore deviant.

This would be less of an issue if our erotic imagination were better behaved, more in line with our public persona. In our internal erotic geography, we all have places that are dear to us. Chances are that at least some of them are places we must sneak into, eluding the watchdog of our conscience. The man who relishes making tender love to his wife has no need for concealment—ditto the woman who fantasizes about a dozen roses from her lover strewn over her bed. Nothing about their romantic aspirations is cause for discomfort or guilt. We should all be so lucky. An imagination peopled with little ladies and gentlemen, so considerate and polite, would easily slip by our internal board of ethics. But the erotic mind is rarely so docile.

What turns us on often collides with our preferred self-image, or with our moral and ideological convictions. Ergo the feminist who longs to be dominated; the survivor of sexual abuse who infuses her personal erotics with her traumatic experiences; the husband who fantasizes about the au pair (the stripper, the masseuse, the porn star) in order to boost his enjoyment with his wife; the mother who finds the skin-to-skin contact with her baby sensuous and, yes, erotic; the wife who masturbates to images of hot sex with the psychopathic boyfriend she knew she was never going to marry; the lover who needs to think about the hunk he spotted at the gym in order to get off with his boyfriend.

We think that there must be something wrong with us for having such prurient thoughts—that this kind of fantasy doesn't belong in the erotic life of the happily married woman, that domination and objectification have no legitimate place in the mind of an upstanding husband and father.

The greater our discomfort with the content of our erotic imagination, the greater the guilt and shame we feel, and the more powerful our internal censors. Ralph has been living with Sharon for fifteen years. By all accounts they are a very happy pair. But soon after they got together, Ralph found himself fantasizing every time they made love: his beloved Sharon kept getting replaced by a seventeen-year-old vixen in a darkened movie theater. For Ralph, his inner life is like a tribal war: the tender lover on one side and the lecherous groper on the other. He confessed one day, "This doesn't sit right with me. I would never touch a seventeen-year-old. I see myself as a decent person, and I can't connect the dots. There's no way I can admit this to Sharon. I can hardly admit it to myself."

In fact, the erotic imagination is fueled by a host of feelings that are far from proper: aggression, raw lust, infantile neediness, power, revenge, selfishness, and jealousy (to name only a few). These feelings, which are all permanent residents of our intimate relations, can threaten the stability of our connection and make love miserable. It is much easier, and often wiser, to banish them to the edge of our imagination, where they can do no harm. In the antechambers of the erotic mind, the rules of propriety are turned on their heads, often invited in for the sole purpose of being trampled. Forbidden frontiers are crossed, gender roles are reversed, modesty is corrupted, and imbalances of power are luxuriously played out, all for the sake of excitement. In fantasy we act out what we dare not do in reality.

Joni and Ray

Joni's lament goes something like this: "Ray thinks I don't like sex. But I do like sex, or at least I used to, I just don't like it so much with him. He doesn't get me sexually, and I can't seem to let him in on it, either. It feels hopeless. I'm only twenty-nine. That's too young to stop having sex."

"Is there a right age to stop having sex?" I ask her. "Later maybe we can pick a date. For now, I'd rather know what is it you want from Ray that you're not getting."

"I want him to be more of a man, and I can't believe I'm saying that out loud." she says, shaking her head. "I don't even know what it means. Like I want him to be some kind of 1950s Neanderthal. But I don't want that. My mother had that. I don't think my father ever asked her what she liked, in the bedroom or out of it. Ray is a mensch. He's a real gentleman, he respects me, and he lets me be. I love how easy our relationship is, but it doesn't do a thing for me sexually."

"What's missing?" I inquire.

Suddenly she leans over and grabs my wrist, not roughly, but with confidence. "This is what I want," she says. Then, tentatively, gently, she brushes my forearm and adds, "This is what I get."

"So he's passive?"

"Not exactly. He initiates sex all the time, but the way he does it makes me crazy. He just sort of raises his eyebrows and goes, 'Hmmm?' It feels like he's asking me, 'Am I going to get laid tonight?' like I'm supposed to take over from there."

"He has a way of approaching you that doesn't say, 'I want you,' as much as 'Do you want me?' Is that it?"

"Yes!" Joni shouts.

I explain that if I'm going to understand what she wants from Ray, first I have to understand what it is she wants sex to provide. "If sex is a quest," I ask her, "what is your Holy Grail?"

Joni is quite forthcoming in disclosing her sexual past: the best experiences she's had, the worst, and what made them so. She gives me a raft of information about the atmosphere she grew up in, her early stirrings, the age she started to masturbate, and the age when she understood what masturbation was. But when I ask her, "What does sex mean to you? What are the feelings that accompany your desire? What do you seek in sex? What do you want to feel? To express? Where do you hold back?" she looks at me, perplexed. "I have no idea," she admits. "No one's ever asked me that before."

All of us invest our erotic encounters with a complex set of needs and expectations. We seek love, pleasure, and validation. Some of us find in sex the perfect venue for rebellion and escape. Others reach for transcendence and ecstasy, even spiritual communion. What I got from Joni was a history of her experience. What I was looking for was a sense of the longings and conflicts she brought to these experiences.

"Can I ask you about your fantasies?" I ask.

Joni pales. "Oh, God. That's so personal. What I do, or what I have done, doesn't seem nearly as embarrassing as what goes on in my mind."

"But that's exactly where I want us to go. I have a sense that if we talk about your fantasies we may be able to get to the heart of what stands between you and Ray."

Over time, and with much coaxing, Joni divulges a fantastic collection of intemperate, luscious, and infinitely detailed erotic tableaux, which she's been constructing since early adolescence. Cowboys, pirates, kings, and concubines parade in endless configurations of carefully wielded power and highly refined surrender. Over the years the plots have changed, but the essence has not. The latest installment takes place on her "husband's" ranch, where she is ritualistically presented to his hired hands as a sexual offering. The night they arrive, she is told to dress for dinner, where she'll be meeting his staff. Her husband (who is, in her characterization, emphatically not Ray) chooses her clothing, an elegant, highly revealing dress and other exquisitely fitting adornments—chandelier earrings, a diamond pendant dangling between her breasts, stiletto heels. He pays attention to every detail of her appearance. After the meal, he asks her to undress for them, so they can appreciate her beauty. She complies; even though she is embarrassed and even humiliated, all this is oddly thrilling. She is completely at their mercy, and makes no attempt to escape. The men are given their own challenge—to anticipate her every desire, and to bring her to heights of sexual ecstasy she has never before known.

"You want to know what I'm afraid of? I'm afraid that I'm a masochist, just like my mother," she tells me.

"How are you a masochist in this story?" I inquire.

"I submit. I'm passive, I'm without my own will. I do what I'm told, and I like being told what to do. What am I doing there, taking orders from men? I resent taking orders from anybody. I can't stand authority, but I get off on submitting to a bunch of cowboys? It makes no fucking sense."

"Actually, it makes quite a lot of sense to me," I tell her.

"Well, would you mind enlightening the rest of us, Doctor?"

I explain that sexual fantasy doesn't work like other fantasies. If people tell me they daydream about a vacation in Tahiti, I believe they want a vacation in Tahiti. The connection between what they fantasize about and what they really want is refreshingly uncomplicated. But sexual fantasies don't reflect reality in the same way. The point about sexual fantasy is that it involves pretending. It's a simulation, a performance—not the real thing, and not necessarily a desire for the real thing. Like dreams and works of art, fantasies are far more than what they appear to be on the surface. They're complex psychic creations whose symbolic content mustn't be translated into literal intent. "Think poetry, not prose," I tell her.

From everything Joni had told me about her relationship with Ray, I didn't think she needed to worry about being a masochist, or even about being passive. The cowboys may be controlling her, but ultimately she is the one controlling the cowboys. She is the author, the producer, the casting agent, the director, and the star of the show. The whole thing is a production staged by her for the purpose of pleasure, not pain. These are worshippers, not sadists. If she were really being forced, she would not be having such a good time. Even though the means is control, her experience is one of care. The convoluted plots are just a safe pathway to pleasure.

When I explain to Joni that her fantasy seems to be more about attention and vulnerability than masochism, her relief is palpable. She is a recovering alcoholic, and so the idea that she has dependency issues comes as no surprise to her. She has been denying her need for support her whole life, even while secretly longing for someone to take care of her. The only thing she's ever felt safe enough to depend on was alcohol, a consistent and reliable friend. More to the point, alcohol never asked for anything in return.

At thirteen Joni applied to boarding school on her own initiative, was accepted, and left home for good. At the time she thought of herself as an ambitious girl. In retrospect, she realizes that this was an attempt to escape the problematic distribution of needs and resources that ruled the family's emotional economy. Over the years she has developed a network of solid friendships that have nurtured her in many ways. But in the end, neither boarding school, nor her career, nor alcohol, nor even her friends have protected her from the inescapable dependency or from the quagmire of vulnerabilities that intimate love entails.

Act II: Enter Ray. In his own words, Ray is a meat-and-potatoes man. He's the happy product of successful male socialization: independent, self-reliant, and able to handle his own problems. He was not like the guys Joni usually dated—struggling, self-absorbed, emotionally undependable, alcoholic artists who weaseled out of relationships by saying things like, "Let's not try to define this; can't we just see where it goes?" and "It's because I like you that I can't be with you." Ray, on the other hand, made it clear that he was interested. He called when he said he would, was never late, and put a lot of thought into planning their dates. "He actually paid attention to what I said. He asked me questions about myself and remembered the answers. I was used to a scene where you can have sex with someone for six months and never even broach the subject of what that might mean or where it might be going. Ray didn't play that game. He liked me and wasn't afraid to say so."

Ray's openness, his consistency, and his emotional generosity brought Joni a sense of peace and security she had never known in a romantic relationship. She found his ability to intuit her needs positively enchanting, and the fact that he seemed to have so few needs of his own was also a plus.

"What an irresistible lure, having a man who can anticipate your needs," I said. "Tell me, how long did it last?"

"Not long enough. I feel like I'm constantly having to ask Ray for everything these days; sometimes I have to ask him twice. I can't stand it," she answers.

"Ah, cowboys to the rescue. You don't even have to ask them once."

Over the course of therapy, I am repeatedly struck by the force of Joni's aversion to any expression of need. There's something extreme about how humiliated and subjugated the need for care leaves her feeling, and I can see how her fantasies of cowboys tap right into this core emotional issue. In her colorful erotic tales, she's able to be at the mercy of others with none of the debilitating powerlessness she dreads. This particular script (and indeed each of her other fantasies) allows her to circumvent the dangers of dependence: the helplessness, the fury, the humiliations. Moreover—and this is important—she is desired for the very qualities that she most loathes about herself in reality. In the refuge of her mind she transforms passivity into erotic delight; power becomes an expression of care, and risk is reunited with safety.

Joni is overcome by the consequences of dependence on all fronts: her own neediness is abject, and the emotional needs of others are likewise overwhelming. She resolves this by peopling her fantasies with caricatures of machismo. These are forceful men who have no weaknesses and need no care. These men don't ask; they take. Joni is thus relieved of the social imperative of female caretaking, and her own carefree sexual greed is liberated.

Behind the Cowboy's Mask

Erotic fantasies have an uncanny ability to resolve more than one issue at a time. While Joni's fantasies certainly speak to her individual conflicts, they also answer a cultural taboo against women's sexuality in general. Massive investments have been made throughout history to ensure that female sexual desire is kept in check. To their credit, women have consistently risen to the challenge of overcoming this taboo. With every new injunction, their imagination has grown more resistant. Consciously, Joni identifies with the women in her stories. But she also created the men, and she has every detail in place. In effect, she plays all the parts. She knows what it means to be a sexual predator: she knows about lust and ruthlessness. Vicariously, through her cowboys, she gets to feel aggression, selfishness, and power—all attributes so wrapped up with masculinity in her mind that they can be expressed only through male characters.

For many women, simulations of forced seduction provide a safe outlet for sexual aggression. Female sexual aggression so contradicts our cultural notions of femininity that we can unleash it only in these imaginary transpositions. Let him, the invented assailant, express the aggression so many women are reluctant to express themselves.

The widespread sexual abuse of women is a chilling backdrop to the now pedestrian rape fantasy, but in these imaginary plots the assault is not real. Few women incorporate a black eye or a split lip into their erotic reveries. The sex therapist Jack Morin makes the point that fantasy rapists are notably nonviolent. In fantasy, violence is subverted by gentleness. Through the gentle man, women can safely experience the joys of "healthy dominance and powerful surrender."

Meanwhile, Back at the Ranch

In my practice I aim to create a sex-friendly place, free of judgment and moralizing, where people can talk safely about their sexuality. Simply doing that—and often it is not so simple at all—can have a profound effect. Sex becomes both a way to illuminate conflicts over intimacy and desire, and a way to begin to heal these destructive splits. Together, Joni and I use the text of her fantasies to address critical issues between her and Ray. Dependency and passivity, aggression, and control were all feelings that she disavowed for years, they had been allowed only in the privacy of her mind. By reclaiming them in therapy she was one step closer to liberating them at home.

Once Joni was no longer held captive by the shame of her fantasies, she became more relaxed and self-accepting. To her surprise, she was able to approach Ray with all sorts of requests and only a modest amount of trepidation. Conversations ensued in which formidable obstacles were revealed to be nothing more than awkward misunderstandings that, through neglect, had snowballed out of control.

For years Ray had assumed that his gentle approach was what Joni wanted. In fact, he thought that was what all women wanted, and he couldn't figure out why asking "What can I do for you?" warranted such an irritated reply: "Nothing!" He had no way of knowing that, for Joni, being taken care of sexually meant abdicating all responsibility and luxuriating in passive dependency, guilt-free. Their dynamics had become absurd, with her rejection triggering his solicitousness, which in turn triggered more rejection.

When Joni invited Ray to be more assertive and self-directed, this was as liberating for him as for her. For the first time, he felt that there was room for a full range of feelings, not just tender ones. Joni was surprised at Ray's positive response to her own new assertiveness. Even claiming her desire to be passive was an unprecedented act of agency on her part. Like many women, she had internalized the powerful message that bold expressions of female sexuality are whorish, unattractive, selfish, and certainly not part of intimate love. "I was afraid that if I told Ray, 'Do this, don't do that, slow down, stay longer, like this, and this, and this,' it would feel emasculating to him."

By deferring to Ray in all matters sexual, by looking to him for expertise and ignoring her own, Joni had fulfilled the age-old feminine mission of preserving her man's ego and shoring up his masculinity. Or so she thought. But her assumptions proved wrong—because Ray gets turned on by her appetite, and even by her demands. For him, having a woman meet him as a sexual equal takes away the burden of guesswork and the persistent insecurity of never being sure he's doing it right. When she is more forthcoming, he doesn't have to worry about her, and he no longer feels diminished by her placating, lukewarm response. Her exuberance gives him permission to make some demands of his own, and to experience unrestrained abandon with the woman he loves.

Joni never did tell Ray the specific content of her fantasies, but unearthing their meaning nonetheless brought about significant changes in their sexual and emotional relationship. Once Joni knew what she was seeking in sex, and once she understood the personal and social barriers that stood in the way of her pleasure, she was able to approach and respond to Ray very differently. To me she said, "Now that I'm clearer about what sex means to me, and how I want to feel in sex, I can talk to Ray about it without having to spell out the fantasy. Although even doing that doesn't seem as scary to me now—there's nothing in there I'm ashamed of or afraid to face."

To Tell or Not to Tell

Some couples get an erotic charge from sharing their fantasies in words or in enactments. Catherine and her husband scheme in naughty complicity when they plan out the details of their lascivious one-acts. This is fun, it's novel, and it allows them to be (and be with) someone new without having to go somewhere else. It creates multiplicity out of monogamy.

But not everyone wants a ticket to this theater of seduction. Disclosure is not a necessary part of working with fantasy. I don't advocate a tell-all approach; not everyone would choose to live in an atmosphere of *True Confessions*. We may like to keep our imaginings to ourselves, not out of shame but out of an inchoate awareness that exposure to bright light will cause them to wither on the vine. Alternatively, we may be wise to dream alone, for we may not be on the same erotic wavelength as our beloved.

Let's take Nat and his girlfriend, Amanda, as an example. Nat's fantasy life isn't tucked away neatly in the privacy of his head; it's evident in the tapes stacked in plain view on his video rack: *Gang Bang 1, Gang Bang 2, Gang Bang 17, Gang Bang 50*. His taste in pornography is unmistakable. He's never felt a need to hide it, but neither has he felt a desire to share it. "It's kind of a fetish for me. I don't think people always understand their fetishes. Why do some people like shoes? I have no clue. I've tried to understand it, but I don't. I'm not being coy. It's been a long-standing thing for me, right back to when I was a teenager, regardless of my actual sex life."

Nat might have coasted along comfortably in his private meanderings were it not for the fact that Amanda is bothered by the tapes. (Still, he must have suspected that leaving them out in plain view would raise this issue.) "I don't get the violence. It scares me. It taps into my own vulnerability as a woman," she says. "I mean, there's something kind of sick about it all, right?" Amanda sees lustful men with absolute power taking advantage of defenseless women. But Nat is watching a very different movie. When I ask him, "Who has the power here?" he is quick to reply, "The woman, without a doubt." For Nat, the turn-on is the insatiable woman, the sexually powerful woman who incorporates several men at once. There is neither force nor hurt associated with his pleasure. "She wants it, and she likes it. If she didn't, it would stop me cold."

Nat's explanations are a relief to Amanda in that they make the movies seem less creepy, but she's still hurt by the fact that the women on the screen are nothing like her. "I can't compete with these women. If this is what he likes, then how can he possibly be satisfied with me?" she asks. When Amanda watches the movies, she thinks only of what they imply about her, not what they convey about Nat, and she feels rejected.

"I do find these women sexy," he admits. "I see a girl walking down the street in a bustier and short leather mini skirt and come-fuck-me boots and, yeah, that turns me on. But do I want to spend the rest of my life with that person? No. Do I want to jeopardize my relationship with you to go fuck that person? No. Have I been attracted to those people in the past, have I fucked those people? Yes. Have I had long-term relationships with any of those people? No. I think I can recognize the difference between something I see as a turn-on versus somebody that I actually love. I think I'm mature enough to handle that concept. My feelings for you are something altogether different."

I invite Amanda to consider that what excites Nat is precisely that the women in his fantasies are not real. It is the very absence of psychological complexity that fuels his arousal. For if these women were real—if they had feelings, needs, insecurities, opinions—an entire closetful of boots wouldn't do it. In these fantasies, complex personalities are substantially narrowed down to get just what he wants from them. The women in his pornographic movies must be sufficiently empty (i.e., objectified) to absorb his imaginary projections and fulfill his needs.

Nat conjures up images of the ravenous succubus. For Joni, it's the cowboys, none too complex themselves. For Daryl it's the lewd passerby on the beach. For Catherine it's her husband in the role of a customer. Our fantasies are often peopled with these personifications of unbridled sexuality. With them we can experience simple enjoyment or irrepressible lust, unfettered by the entangling emotions of adult intimacy. These welcome strangers help us sidestep the ambiguities of desire and the contingencies of love. Though they live side by side with love, they're not a substitute for the real thing.

Heterosexual pornography, predominantly produced by and for men, concerns itself almost exclusively with what the sociologist Anthony Giddens calls "low emotion, high intensity sex." In part, it meets the need of many men to compartmentalize their sexual and emotional lives, and to separate their secure relationships from their rash urges. But it also serves an additional purpose not immediately apparent. While opponents of porn focus primarily on the aggression and violence of male sexuality, Giddens makes the point that the male potency displayed in these stories is a manifest reassurance against male insecurities—sexual and other. The female characters in much pornography (themselves invulnerable) neutralize male vulnerability because they are always fully responsive and fully satisfied. The man never suffers from inadequacy, because the woman is in a state of ecstatic bliss that is entirely his doing. She confirms his virility.

While Nat listened to my rudimentary deconstruction of pornography, I had the sense that he would just as soon have been anywhere else. He did not welcome the idea that *Gang Bang 47* was really about male sexual insecurity. But he did identify with the need for an emotion-free zone where sex could be unencumbered and raw, and where all vulnerabilities, inadequacies, and dependencies—his and hers—might be temporarily suspended.

Had the tapes not been out there, I might not have initiated this level of discussion about Nat's viewing habits. For one thing, Nat and Amanda had not been with each other long; they were still anchoring their life together, negotiating many aspects of their relationship. I sensed that Amanda's insecurities, prejudices, and aesthetic differences would make it difficult for her to hear about his private turn-ons in a way that didn't threaten her.

For his part, Nat was not especially responsive to Amanda's sensibilities. He was cavalier about the effect all these tapes were having on her, and (contrary to his own objections) he was being a bit coy about not understanding what it all meant. His argument that he loved her too much to be able to eroticize her that way was too glib. Exposing one's inner erotic life demands more sensitivity and tact than Nat exhibited. Likewise, entering the fantasy world of our partner requires more sense of separateness than Amanda was able to muster.

Some people get off on peeking behind the curtain of their partner's secret imaginings; for others, this is a disaster. It not only fails to enrich but actually hurts their erotic complicity. Inviting someone into the recesses of our erotic mind is risky. When the fantasy is poorly received it can be devastating. But when it's received in a way that makes us feel recognized and accepted, it can be richly affirming. While the fantasy itself may not be an intimate scenario, its disclosure expresses and fosters deep love and trust.

At the same time, entering the erotic mindscape of another requires an effort of understanding and a considerable degree of emotional separateness. We may not like what we hear; we may not find it sexy. This level of compassionate objectivity is not easy to achieve, especially with regard to desire. If our partner is aroused by something foreign to us, something other, the temptation is to judge first and ask questions later, if at all. What begins as an open inquiry can rapidly degenerate into a mutually defensive withdrawal. When the erotic mind senses criticism, it goes into hiding. No longer private, it becomes secretive.

I am a proponent of privacy, and I prefer a cautious approach in matters of sexual self-disclosure. Exploring one's eroticism is not synonymous with making it public; and acknowledging need not mean detailed sharing. There are many ways to bring our erotic selves into our intimate relationships; they don't all require words or literal exposés. How to go about it will depend on the particular relationship and the compatibility of the partners.

Our cultural taboos about erotic fantasy are so strong that for many people the very idea of discussing it creates anxiety and shame. Yet fantasies are maps of our psychological and cultural preoccupations; exploring them can lead to greater self-awareness, an essential step in creating change. When we cordon off our erotic interiors, we are left with sex that is truncated, devoid of vibrancy, and not particularly intimate. What people fail to see is that dull, boring sexual relationships are often a consequence of shutting down the imagination in just this way.

Our erotic imagination is an exuberant expression of our aliveness, and one of the most powerful tools we have for keeping desire alive. Giving voice to our fantasies can liberate us from the many personal and social obstacles that stand in the way of pleasure. Understanding what our fantasies do for us will help us understand what it is we're seeking, sexually and emotionally. In our erotic daydreams, we find the energy that keeps us passionately awake to our own sexuality.

10

The Shadow of the Third

Rethinking Fidelity

Q: Are there any secrets to long-lasting relationships?
A: Infidelity. Not the act itself, but the threat of it. For Proust, an
injection of jealousy is the only thing capable of rescuing a
relationship ruined by habit.

— *Alain de Botton,* How Proust Can Change Your Life

The bonds of wedlock are so heavy that it takes two to carry them,
sometimes three.

— *Alexandre Dumas*

THE TALMUD, THE GREAT COMPILATION of rabbinic tradition, tells the
following parable. Every night, Rabbi Bar Ashi would prostrate
himself before the merciful God and beg to be saved from the evil
urge. His wife, overhearing him, would think, "It's been a number
of years since he has withdrawn from me. What makes him say
that?" So one day, as he is studying in the garden, she dresses herself up as Haruta and meets him there. (Haruta was the name of the
quintessential prostitute in ancient Babylon. The word also means
"freedom" in Hebrew.)

"Who are you?" he asks.

"I am Haruta," she answers.

"I want you," he commands.

"Bring me the pomegranate on the uppermost branch," she demands in turn.

He brings her the pomegranate, and takes her.

When he returns home his wife is tending the fire. He rises, and tries to throw himself in. She asks, "Why are you doing so?"

"Because thus and thus happened," he confesses.

"But it was I," she responds.

"I, however, intended the forbidden."

Monolithic Monogamy

The moment two people become a couple, they begin to deal with boundaries—what is in and what is out. You choose one among all others, then draw the lines around your blissful union. Now the questions begin. What am I free to do alone and what do I have to share? Do we go to bed at the same time? Will you be joining my family at every Thanksgiving? Sometimes we negotiate these arrangements explicitly, but more often we proceed by trial and error. You see how much you can get away with before tripwiring on sensitivities. Why didn't you ask me to join you? I thought we'd travel together. A look, a comment, a bruised silence—these are the clues we have to interpret. We intuit how often to see each other, how often to talk, and how much sharing is expected. We sift through our respective friendships and decide how important they're allowed to be now that we have each other. We sort out ex-lovers—do we know about them, talk about them, see them? Whether aboveboard or below, we delineate zones of privacy as well as zones of togetherness.

The mother of all boundaries, the reigning queen, is fidelity, for she more than any other confirms our union. Traditionally, monogamy was viewed as one sexual partner for life, like swans and wolves. Today, it has come to mean having one sexual partner at a time. (As it turns out, even swans and wolves only appear to be monogamous.) The woman who marries, divorces, is single for a while, has several lovers, remarries, divorces, then marries for a third time can nonetheless meet the criteria for monogamy provided that she remains sexually exclusive within each relationship. Yet a man who is committed to the same woman for fifty years, but allows himself a one-night tryst in the fifteenth year, is readily consigned to the category of the infidel. If you've cheated, you've cheated.

As Bob Dylan sang "The times they are a-changing." In the past fifty years we have opened ourselves to a wealth of new marital and family configurations. We can have straight, gay, or transgender marriages. We can have domestic partnerships. We can be single parents, stepparents, adoptive parents, or child-free. Successive marriages and blended families are common. We can cohabitate and never marry, or we can be in a commuter marriage with only brief stints under one roof. Finely attuned to the fragility of matrimony, we now have prenuptial agreements and no-fault divorce. All these arrangements have redefined boundaries both within the couple and between the couple and the outside world. Yet, however elastic our attitudes toward marriage, we remain unflinching in our insistence on monogamy. With few exceptions—movie stars, aging hippies, swingers—the borders we draw around sexual exclusivity remain rigid.

Our love affair with monogamy arguably comes at some cost. The Brazilian family therapist Michele Scheinkman says, "American culture has great tolerance for divorce—where there is a total breakdown of the loyalty bond and painful effects for the whole family—but it is a culture with no tolerance for sexual infidelity." We would rather kill a relationship than question its structure.

So entrenched is our faith in monogamy that most couples, particularly heterosexual couples, rarely broach the subject openly.

They have no need to discuss what's a given. Even those who are otherwise willing to probe sexuality in all its permutations are often reluctant to negotiate the hard lines around exclusivity. Monogamy has an absolute quality. According to this way of thinking, you can't be mostly monogamous, or 98 percent monogamous, or periodically nonmonogamous. Discussing fidelity implies that it's open to discussion, no longer an imperative. The prospect of betrayal is too dark, so we avoid the subject with practiced denial. We fear that the smallest chink in our armor will let in Sodom and Gomorrah.

Despite a 50 percent divorce rate for first marriages and 65 percent the second time around; despite the staggering frequency of affairs; despite the fact that monogamy is a ship sinking faster than anyone can bail it out, we continue to cling to the wreckage with absolute faith in its structural soundness.

Finding the One

Historically, monogamy was an externally imposed system of control over women's reproduction. "Which child is mine? Who gets the cows when I die?" Fidelity, as a mainstay of patriarchal society, was about lineage and property; it had nothing to do with love. Today, particularly in the West, it has everything to do with love. When marriage shifted from a contractual arrangement to a matter of the heart, faithfulness became a mutual expression of love and commitment. Once a social prohibition directed at women, fidelity is now a personal choice for both sexes. Conviction has replaced convention.

These days, we are our own matchmakers. No longer obligated to marry who we must, we set out with a new ideal of what we want, and we want plenty. Our desiderata still include everything the traditional family was meant to provide—security, children, property, respectability—but now we also want our Joe to love us, to desire us, to be interested in us. We should be confidants, best friends, and passionate lovers. Modern marriage promises us that there is one person out there with whom all this is possible if we can just find her. So tenaciously do we hold to the idea that marriage is for everything that the disenchanted opt for divorce or affairs not because they question the institution, but because they think they chose the wrong person with whom to reach this nirvana. Next time they'll choose better. The focus is always on the object of our love, not on our capacity to love. Hence the psychologist Erich Fromm makes the point that we think it's easy to love, but hard to find the right person. Once we've found "the one," we will need no one else.

The exclusiveness we seek in monogamy has roots in our earliest experience of intimacy with our primary caretakers. The feminist psychoanalyst Nancy Chodorow writes, "This primary tendency, I shall be loved always, everywhere, in every way, my whole body, my whole being—without any criticism, without the slightest effort on my part—is the final aim of all erotic striving." In our adult love we seek to recapture the primordial oneness we felt with Mom. The baby knows no separateness. Once upon a time, there was one person whose only role was to be there for us. In the ecstatic communion between mother and child, there is no gap. To the newborn the mother is everything, all at once, inseparable, unbounded: her skin, her breast, her voice, her smile, it is all for him. As a pink-bottomed baby, we were full and fulfilled, and somewhere deep inside we've never forgotten that Eden. Those of us who didn't know this idyllic state—those with mothers who were unavailable, inconsistent, absent, or selfish—are often even more determined to find the perfect partner.

The question remains: isn't the oneness we strive to restore itself a fantasy? For the child, Mom is the be-all and end-all, but the mother has always known other people. She even has a jealous lover, the father. As it turns out, Mom was never totally faithful—not even once upon a time.

So the specter of betrayal is there from the beginning. We grow up with it. The isolating conditions of modern life only amplify the rumbling insecurity that hides in the background of our romantic possessiveness. Fear of loss and fear of abandonment tighten our grip on fidelity. In a culture where everything is disposable and downsizing confirms just how replaceable we really are, our need to feel secure in our primary relationship is all the greater. The smaller we feel in the world, the more we need to shine in the eyes of our partner. We want to know that we matter, and that, for at least one person, we are irreplaceable. We long to feel whole, to rise above the prison of our solitude.

Perhaps this is why our insistence on sexual exclusivity is absolute. Because adult sexual love momentarily reenacts that most primitive form of early fusion—the merging of bodies, the nipple that fills our entire mouth and leaves us completely satiated—the thought of our beloved with another is cataclysmic. Sex, we feel, is the ultimate betrayal.

Monogamy, it follows, is the sacred cow of the romantic ideal, for it is the marker of our specialness: I have been chosen and others renounced. When you turn your back on other loves, you confirm my uniqueness; when your hand or mind wanders, my importance is shattered. Conversely, if I no longer feel special, my own hands and mind tingle with curiosity. The disillusioned are prone to roam. Might someone else restore my significance?

The Matrimonial Jackpot

Doug met his first wife in college. They were good friends, but their sex life was never particularly interesting. Eventually it, and the marriage, fizzled out. He went on to have a few passionate relationships that left him sexually invigorated but emotionally spent. Then he met Zoë, an energetic and joyful CGI artist with what he calls a "low neurotic quotient." He goes on, "She was one of a kind. Down-to-earth, practical, and wild in bed. I thought I'd hit the matrimonial jackpot."

Several years into the marriage, she has stopped responding to him so enthusiastically. She still has a lot of energy, but much of it is directed elsewhere. The kids demand her attention. Animation saps her creativity. And her size X-L family—her parents, her five sisters, and all their kids—are the hub of her social life. Doug feels unnoticed. Without sex to distinguish him among the cast of characters in his wife's busy life, he feels increasingly irrelevant, like an extra.

In the ensuing years, Doug's growing irritability is punctuated by brief flashes of seductive instigation. He whisks Zoë away on romantic weekends, carefully selects the weekly DVDs, buys earrings because she fancies dangling baubles. For the most part, Zoë is game. But the more Doug pursues her, the more he realizes how essential his effort is, and this depresses him. Despite all the kindling, he never manages to light the roaring blaze he needs. The more he tries to fill the gap, the emptier he feels. His eyes begin to wander, and when they finally focus, it's not on Zoë; it's on Naomi.

This striking redheaded retail buyer isn't subtle about expressing her attraction to Doug. She finds excuses to go into his office, and once there, she lingers. She's impressed by how well he handled their boss; she likes that suit; are those new glasses? A sandwich turns into a drink turns into a five-year affair. The sex is fiery, but that's not what the affair is about. It's about the abundance of attention, and the exhilaration of the illicit. With Naomi, who never lacks for male attention, Doug is irresistible. She misses him on the weekends; she's jealous about his other life. And while her possessiveness drains him, and is sometimes annoying, it also confirms exactly how important he is.

When Doug comes to see me, he can barely manage the contradictions in his life. His marriage, which is supposed to be monogamous, is not. His affair, which is de facto nonmonogamous, has just ended because he couldn't meet Naomi's demand for fidelity. "The whole thing is insane," he tells me. "Naomi wanted me to stop having sex with Zoë, which I told her I couldn't do. So she started seeing someone else, and now they're talking about marriage. She's refusing to have sex with me, and she's completely secretive about her relationship with Evan. I'm so jealous I'm obsessed. The thought of her in the arms of another guy makes me nuts."

"I hope the irony isn't lost on you," I tell him. "You demand fidelity in the very place that's defined by infidelity."

"Yeah, but that's her infidelity, not mine," he answers.

"Oh, yes, I forgot there's a double standard. She and Zoë are both expected to remain faithful to you while you remain faithful to neither?"

"Something like that, yeah. Not a very fair arrangement, I know. Believe me, I'm not proud."

"So why didn't you leave Zoë?" I ask. "If you had all this with Naomi, why didn't you follow the burning bush, the fire that never consumes?"

"I love Zoë," Doug says, shocked at the implications of what I've just said. "I've never really wanted to leave my marriage. I have a good thing with Zoë, and I don't want to live away from my kids. Anyway, Naomi and I married? That would be a disaster."

"So this wasn't an exit affair. Maybe more like a stabilizer, where the third person helps keep the other two in place?"

"I don't know. Maybe. The point is that I didn't think. I just did it. I followed my gut, and now I feel like shit."

Unpacking the Affair

On some level, I think Doug would like me to confirm that indeed he has done something terribly wrong. He has betrayed his vows, a moral offense in black and white. But wholesale condemnation too easily distracts us from the real issues behind his behavior. I prefer a morally neutral stance that leaves us free to explore the meaning of the affair rather than the ethics of it. Once Doug understands the motives that drove him into Naomi's arms, he'll be able to draw his own conclusions, both about what he did and about what he wants to do henceforth.

People stray for many reasons—tainted love, revenge, unfulfilled longings, plain old lust. At times an affair is a quest for intensity, or a rebellion against the confines of matrimony. Transgression is an aphrodisiac, and sometimes secrets are a source of autonomy, or a backlash against lack of privacy. What could be more titillating than a whispered phone call in the bathroom? Finally, the harried mom can feel like a woman again; her lover knows nothing about the broken Lego set or the plumber who failed to show up for the second time.

An illicit liaison can be catastrophic, but it can also be a liberation, a source of strength, a healing. Frequently it is all these things at once. When the intimacy is gone, when we no longer talk, when we haven't been touched in years, we are more vulnerable to the kindness of strangers. When the kids are young and needy, extramarital appreciation can feel like a tonic. When they're older and gone, empty nesters may seek replenishment elsewhere. If our health fails us, or if we've just been visited by death, we may experience outbursts of dissatisfaction, a cry for something better. Some affairs are acts of resistance; others happen when we offer no resistance at all. Straying can sound an alarm for the marriage, signaling an urgent need to pay attention. Or it can be the death knell that follows a relationship's last, gasping breath.

I question the widespread view that infidelity is always a symptom of deeper problems in a relationship. Affairs are motivated by myriad forces; not all of them are directly related to flaws in the marriage. As it happens, plenty of adulterers are reasonably content in their relationships. So was Doug. But he wanted more. He couldn't articulate what it was exactly, only that it had something to do with more frequent sex.

Together, Doug and I explore the anatomy of his passion, and I come to understand what needs are met in his tumultuous relationship with Naomi. For him, sex is a place of emotional nourishment and a sanctuary. It is love incarnate. Through sex he reaches an egoless oblivion that makes him feel at one with the world. Passion grants Doug ultimate relief from the unbearable aloneness of being. "It's like I'm gone; it washes everything out. That kind of absolute focus, total attention, somehow releases me from myself. I stop thinking, the sensation washes up my spine, through my brain, and out. But there's no observing of what's going on." Lovemaking is all-encompassing. With Naomi, Doug is able to maintain this high-octane, transcendent sex. In part, this is because erotically they are made of the same cloth. But, more important, the very structure of their affair, and of all affairs, lends itself to passion.

Affairs are risky, dangerous, and labile, all elements that fuel excitement. In the self-contained universe of adulterous love you are secluded from the rest of the world, and your bond is strengthened by the secrecy that surrounds it. Never exposed to broad daylight, the spell of the other is preserved. There's no need to worry that your friends won't like him, since nobody knows about him. Affairs unfold in the margins of our lives, and are luxuriously free of the dental appointments, taxes, and bills.

Then there are barriers to overcome. To see each other, you have to make an effort, sometimes a huge one. There are hoops to jump through, schedules to juggle, locations to secure, excuses to invent. And all that unflagging zeal repeatedly affirms the lovers' importance to each other. Seen in this light, Doug's transgression was an attempt to recapture what he once had with his wife and could not live without: a sense of importance, a relief from loneliness, and a feeling of robustness.

You Can Go Home Again

By the time the affair ends, Doug's marriage is down to the bare bones. Doug and Zoë are cordial, respectful, even occasionally affectionate, but emotionally they have flatlined. They have grown accustomed to vagueness regarding his repeated absences. His overtures are few and far between, and he is distracted. He is afraid of unintentionally disclosing something with a slip of the tongue; his secrecy is taking up more and more acreage in their marriage, leaving him with few subjects he can freely discuss with Zoë: the kids, the president, and the weather.

As we unravel what sparked Doug's affair with Naomi, it becomes clear to me why he chose not to fight for her but instead to stay with his wife. Zoë is terra firma. At the same time, her ability to keep things in perspective gives her a certain ease; it's not hard for her to sleep through the night, or to get up in the morning. Zoë doesn't seek passion. She is rarely swept away. With Naomi, Doug may have found the single missing piece, but with Zoë he has the rest of the puzzle.

Doug and I discuss how his ideal of marriage holds up to the reality of his own particular union. He wants heat and warmth in the same place. He wants the kitchen table to be an altar of carnal merging at night, and a sunny breakfast nook for pancakes with the kids the next morning. But Doug will probably never experience with Zoë the same intensity he has had with Naomi. Affairs have their own brand of passion. Secrecy, torment, guilt, transgression, danger, risk, and jealousy are highly combustible, a Molotov cocktail, an erotic explosion far too threatening in a home with children.

As Doug becomes clearer about what he can reasonably expect from his marriage, a new set of questions arises. What are his options now that he has chosen to stay? Can he recognize his desires without having to act on them? Will he continue to negotiate monogamy privately, without Zoë's knowledge, as is typical in affairs; or might he opt for a more open discussion of the sexual boundaries around their marriage? Must he disclose the affair in order to reconnect with his wife? What can he do with his guilt?

The answers change every day. Last week, it seemed as if he would never be able to look her in the eye unless he came clean. Today, it seems that the most loving thing he can do is to keep his mess to himself. "Do I break her heart just to ease my conscience? Sometimes I think she's known all along, and the only reason she hasn't left me is because I've kept my mouth shut. At least this way she gets to hold on to her dignity."

Most American couples therapists believe that affairs must be disclosed if intimacy is to be rebuilt. This idea goes hand in hand with our model of intimate love, which celebrates transparency—having no secrets, telling no lies, sharing everything. In fact, some people condemn the deception even more than the transgression: "It's not that you cheated, it's that you lied to me!" To the American way of thinking, respect is bound up with honesty, and honesty is essential to personal responsibility. Hiding, dissimulation, and other forms of deception amount to disrespect. You lie only to those beneath you—children, constituents, employees.

In other cultures, respect is more likely to be expressed with gentle untruths that aim at preserving the partner's honor. A protective opacity is preferable to telling truths that might result in humiliation. Hence concealment not only maintains marital harmony but also is a mark of respect. Informed by my own cultural influences, I defer to Doug's decision to remain silent, and at the same time I encourage him to pursue other ways to reconnect with his wife. His marriage has been on "pause" for a long time; now he needs to push the "play" button.

Doug reinvests in his relationship with Zoë. With more time on his hands, and being generally more available, he begins to redirect his abundant resources toward his wife. She feigns surprise at the sudden return of her Odysseus, but beneath her wisecracking "Howdy Stranger" attitude, Doug knows that she is relieved. I encourage him to pump up his involvement with the kids, the house, and the social calendar, hoping that relieving Zoë of some domestic burdens may open her to the erotic.

In his attempts to be more forthcoming, Doug even asks Zoë if she ever finds herself attracted to other men. Her answer is elusive, "Maybe I do. Maybe I don't. What's it to you?" This leaves him slightly rattled. "When someone is as wrapped up in secrecy as you've been," I remark, "it's easy to imagine that you're the mysterious one, the rebel, and she's Penelope sitting at her loom, waiting for you to come home. So maybe she has a few secrets of her own, fantasies of men who can give her what you can't."

Marriage is imperfect. We start with a desire for oneness, and then we discover our differences. Our fears are aroused by the prospect of all the things we're never going to have. We fight. We withdraw. We blame our partners for failing to make us whole. We look elsewhere. Sadly, too many of us stay stuck in this place until we're bald or gray. Others mourn the loss of the dream, then come to terms with the choice they made. Love is anchored in acceptance. When Doug comes to know himself, and to recognize Zoë for who she is, he can finally turn their differences into riches.

The Shadow of the Third

At the boundary of every couple lives the third. He's the high school sweetheart whose hands you still remember, the pretty cashier, the handsome fourth-grade teacher you flirt with when you pick your son up at school. The smiling stranger on the subway is the third. So, too, are the stripper, the porn star, and the sex worker, whether touched or untouched. He is the one a woman fantasizes about when she makes love to her husband. Increasingly, she can be found on the Internet. Real or imagined, embodied or not, the third is the fulcrum on which a couple balances. The third is the manifestation of our desire for what lies outside the fence. It is the forbidden.

The affair is the third, but so, too, is the wife at home. Naomi is the hidden shadow in Doug's marriage, but Zoë lives at the center of the affair. The lovers' jealousy depends on the presence of the spouse. Without the betrothed, all the possessiveness, passion, and insanity of fevered lovers will simply go limp. Perhaps this is why so few affairs last after the marriage that inspired them dissolves. The true test of love in an affair begins only when the obstacle is removed.

All relationships live in the shadow of the third, for it is the other that solders our dyad. In his book *Monogamy*, Adam Phillips writes, "The couple is a resistance to the intrusion of the third, but in order for it to last it is indispensable to have enemies. That is why the monogamous can't live without them. When we are two, we are together. In order to form a couple, we need to be three."

What then is a couple to do? Many of the patients I meet simply refuse to acknowledge the third. They're drawn by the lure of oneness, which insists that there is no need for others. Perfect love is sufficient unto itself. So fragile is this fusion that the presence of another, even in fantasy, is powerful enough to shatter it.

This is poignantly illustrated in Stanley Kubrick's film *Eyes Wide Shut*. Bill and Alice have just returned from a lavish black-tie Christmas party that has sparked a conversation about sex. Bill has always assumed that Alice, like him, is essentially incapable of infidelity. "You're my wife and my child's mother and I'm sure of you. You'd never be unfaithful. I'm sure of you." Alice, outraged at his presumption and emboldened by a joint they have just smoked, decides to enlighten him. She describes in agonizing detail just how powerful the presence of the other can be, even when it is nothing more than a mirage. She tells him of her febrile fantasy about a naval officer she desired from a distance. They never met; nonetheless, his instant hold on her was so strong she would have given up everything if he'd only asked. She also says that this happened on a day when she and Bill had just made love, and Bill had never been dearer to her.

Bill is devastated by his wife's revelation, and he spends the rest of the film trying to avenge the betrayal and restore order to his broken world. What struck me is that, for Bill, a fantasy could generate the same sense of violation as an actual affair.

Bill is like many of the partners I meet. His security rests not only on what Alice does but also on what she thinks. Her fantasies are proof of her freedom and separateness, and that scares him. The third points to other possibilities, choices we didn't make, and in this way it's bound up with our freedom. Laura Kipnis says, "What is more anxiogenic than a partner's freedom, which might mean the freedom not to love you, or to stop loving you, or to love someone else, or to become a different person than the one who once pledged to love you always and now … perhaps doesn't?" If she can think about others, she might love others, and that is intolerable.

Fortress Love

The menace of the third is intrinsic to the experience of love, and even the most controlling marriage may not be able to allay our anxieties. Nevertheless, many of us do try. "You were with that guy for a while. What were you talking about?" "You spend a lot of time on the computer. Is it all work?" "Where have you been?" "Who was there?" "Did you miss me?" Many of our inquiries hover at the border between intimacy and intrusiveness. We want to know, but we don't want to be too obvious. We say that we ask because we care, but often it's because we're afraid.

So we set up rules and hope our partners will comply, and in this way we preemptively secure faithfulness by keeping a tight leash. Desire is insubordinate; actions are susceptible to reason and so are easier to control. You're not allowed to have close personal friends of the opposite sex. You can't go to a movie with so-and-so unless other people are there. No videos we can't watch together. No strip clubs, except for bachelor parties. No male dancers. That dress is too revealing. You can't reminisce fondly about exes, and you certainly can't see them alone when they pass through town. When our anxiety is too much for us, we fall back on more primitive means of control: we spy. We check credit card statements, the browser's "back" button, the gas tank, the cell phone, scavenging for information. But these strategies invariably fall short. The interrogations, the injunctions, and even the forensic evidence fail to assuage our fundamental fear of our partner's freedom. Our beloved might desire someone else.

Trouble looms when monogamy is no longer a free expression of loyalty but a form of enforced compliance. Excessive monitoring can set the stage for what Stephen Mitchell calls "acts of exuberant defiance." When the third is denied, some people decide to negotiate it privately. Affairs, online encounters, strip clubs, and sex on business trips are common transgressions that establish psychological distance from an overbearing relationship. When the third is exiled to somewhere, only permitted outside the marriage, that is where he is sought.

The Invincible We

In principle we understand that we each deserve privacy, though in practice this matter is a bit trickier. The psychologist Janet Reibstein notes that our companionate, romantic model of marriage, which stresses togetherness and honesty, "is much better at spelling out the criteria for intimacy than those for autonomy." The emphasis is on building closeness, not on sustaining individuality. My patients who adhere closely to this ethos of intimacy wind up feeling that their individual aspirations, or those of their partner, are no longer legitimate. The invincible *we* supersedes the puny *I*.

Niv was frustrated by his girlfriend's early bedtime. "She's a dancer and she goes to sleep at nine o'clock at night. I can't fall asleep that early, so I just lie there." When I ask him if he ever goes out with his friends after she's gone to bed, he's astonished. "I can do that?" The idea of doing that—or even of asking—had never occurred to him. Leila and Mario have been steady dance partners since raves were hip. But when she starts dating Angela, who has two left feet and can't stand loud music, she becomes uncomfortable about her weekly date with Mario. She doesn't want to hurt Angela.

Armed with an ideology of love that advocates togetherness, we are awkward about pursuing autonomy. This is especially true of the individuality of our desire. Even couples who grant one another considerable space elsewhere—separate vacations, nights out on the town, close friends of the opposite sex—grapple with the idea that they might have an erotic life independent of each other. I'm not talking about extramarital sex. I'm talking about a sexual self that is discrete, that generates its own images, responds to others, and is delighted when it gets turned on unexpectedly. It is all these contingencies of desire that I bring to bear on my work with couples.

Monogamous Marriage in a Promiscuous Society

Generally, the role of therapists is to challenge the cultural status quo. We regularly encourage our patients to examine their assumptions about what's normal, acceptable, and expected. Yet sexual boundaries are one of the few areas where therapists seem to mirror the dominant culture. Monogamy is the norm, and sexual fidelity is considered to be mature, committed, and realistic. Nonmonogamy, even consensual nonmonogamy, is suspect. It points to a lack of commitment or a fear of intimacy. It undermines the couple.

As one of my colleagues firmly stated, "Open marriage doesn't work. Thinking you can do it is totally naive. We tried it in the seventies and it was a disaster." "That may be so, but the closed marriage is hardly a guarantee against disaster," I cautioned. "And the monogamous ideal, which a decent chunk of married folks don't live up to, may be no less naive. If anything, it seems to invite transgressions that are excruciatingly painful." My colleague, an excellent family therapist, was nevertheless taking an all-or-nothing approach to fidelity. In this view, emotional commitment demands sexual exclusivity, and brooks no gradations.

Yet we live in a world that offers us little help with staying put or making do. In our consumer culture, we always want the next best thing: the latest, the newest, the youngest. Failing that, we at least want more: more intensity, more variety, more stimulation. We seek instant gratification and are increasingly intolerant of any frustration. Nowhere are we encouraged to be satisfied with what we have, to think, "This is good. This is enough." Sex is part and parcel of this economy—some people might even say that sex propels it. That dress, that car, those shoes, this lotion, a new tattoo, buns of steel, all carry the promise of a more sexually fulfilled life. We are convinced that sexual gratification and personal happiness go hand in hand. Earthly delights are everywhere, a veritable banquet, and we feel entitled to join the feast. No wonder people often feel restless in marriage. The fantasy of infinite variety is thwarted by commitment.

This isn't a justification of infidelity, or an endorsement. Temptation has existed since Eve bit the apple, but so, too, have injunctions against it. The Catholic church is expert not only in avoiding temptation but also in meting out penance for those we couldn't resist. What's different today is not the desires themselves but the fact that we feel obligated to pursue them—at least until we tie the knot, when we're suddenly expected to renounce all we've been encouraged to want. Monogamy stands alone, like the Dutch boy with his finger in the dike, trying to hold back a flood of unbridled licentiousness.

Inviting the Shadow

Some couples choose not to ignore the lure of the forbidden. Instead, they subvert its power by inviting it in. "I would never want him to be unfaithful, but knowing it's possible keeps me sexually interested in him." "Pretending there are no handsome men in the world doesn't make my relationship safer and certainly doesn't make it more honest." "My girlfriend is beautiful. Men are always coming on to her. The way she laughs it off makes me feel great; she keeps picking me." These couples share fantasies, read erotica together, or reminisce about the past. They admit that, yes, the delivery man was hot. So was the computer tech, the salesman at Barney's, your neurologist, the neighbor's wife.

Selena and Max have license to flirt but draw the line at realizing the possibilities. "We're both gluttons for attention. I get a real ego boost when someone hits on me, especially now that I have a kid. And when someone hits on Max? Forget it. I feel like I'm going home with the prom king." Max and Selena like to play with possessiveness, but both are dead certain of the rules of the game.

When Elsa returns from a conference, Gerard is always curious about whom she met. "Was there anyone interesting? Did you tell him about your fantastic husband? And were you flirting while you were raving about me?"

Wendy has always known that George has a weakness for blonds. So last Thursday she decided to be one for the day. She donned a platinum wig and a trench coat and showed up unannounced at the building site to take him to lunch. He says, "Great. The guys are going to think I'm having an affair." Wendy doesn't miss a beat: "Let them be jealous."

These couples, in their own ways, have chosen to acknowledge the possibility of the third: the recognition that our partner has his or her own sexuality, replete with fantasies and desires that aren't necessarily about us. When we validate one another's freedom within the relationship, we're less inclined to search for it elsewhere. In this sense, inviting the third goes some way toward containing its volatility, not to mention its appeal. It is no longer a shadow but a presence, something to talk about openly, joke about, play with. When we can tell the truth safely, we are less inclined to keep secrets.

Rather than inhibiting a couple's sexuality, recognizing the third has a tendency to add spice, not least because it reminds us that we do not own our partners. We should not take them for granted. In uncertainty lies the seed of wanting. In addition, when we establish psychological distance, we, too, can peek at our partner with the admiring eyes of a stranger, noticing once again what habit has prevented us from seeing. Finally, renouncing others reaffirms our choice. He is the one I want. We admit our roving desires, yet push them back. We flirt with them, all the while keeping them at a safe distance. Perhaps this is another way of looking at maturity: not as passionless love, but as love that knows of other passions not chosen.

Inviting the Third

There are a lot of ways to invite the third into a relationship that don't include extramarital sex, and a few that do. For most people, the mention of sexually open relationships sets off the red warning lights. Few subjects having to do with committed love evoke such a visceral response. What if she falls in love with him? What if he never comes back? The idea that you can love one person and have sex with another with impunity makes us shudder. We fear that transgressing one limit can lead to the potential breach of all limits. We conjure up images of chaos: promiscuity, orgies, debauchery. Against this decadence, being a couple is the only barricade. It protects us from our impulses. It is our best defense against unbridled animality.

Adam Phillips makes the point that "monogamy is a kind of moral nexus, a keyhole through which we can spy on our preoccupations." A number of thorny questions arise in discussion of consensual nonmonogamy. Is emotional commitment always bound to sexual exclusivity? Can we love more than one person at the same time? Is sex ever "just sex?" Are men more naturally prone to roam than women? These questions perhaps top the list, but there are more. Is jealousy an expression of love or a sign of insecurity? Why are we eager to share our friends, but demand exclusivity from our lover? I don't pretend to have an answer to these questions. I do believe, however, that we can benefit from taming our romantic nostalgia in order to ponder them seriously.

Even our most entrenched beliefs about sexuality are susceptible to revision. We once shunned premarital sex and homosexuality; they are now more or less accepted in most circles. In recent years, a small group of men and women have taken on monogamy as the next big battle in their personal fight for sexual emancipation.

Joan and Hiro describe having two types of sex: sex for love and sex for fun. The latter they reserve for their annual trip to a swingers' convention in Las Vegas. They tell me that it has done wonders for their sex life as well as for their intimacy. Despite how they may appear, Joan and Hiro are champions of the marital ideals they seem to be defying. They don't question the institution of marriage. In fact, they seek to preserve it. They value togetherness, honesty, and sharing. Even fidelity is upheld in their arrangement. Joan and Hiro have effectively neutralized the threat of infidelity by channeling it into their relationship. And, as the anthropologist Katherine Frank wryly notes, "What happens in Vegas stays in Vegas." Swinging is a form of consensual adultery. It also accords equal freedom to both partners.

Eric and Jaxon are also fans of recreational sex, and in the ten years they've been together they've always made a distinction between emotional loyalty and sexual exclusivity within their commitment. "Right from the start we talked about sex with other men. We're open about it. For us, the real commitment is the emotional one. Sex outside the relationship isn't a deal-breaker. I guess you could call us emotionally monogamous, sexually promiscuous."

Arlene, sixteen years older than Jenna, explains, "I know sex matters, it's just not so important to me anymore. And the older I get, the less I care." Jenna feels she's in her prime, and isn't ready for early retirement. They've agreed that when Jenna goes on location for a shoot, she's allowed to have her fun provided she doesn't forget where her priorities lie. When I ask Arlene if she isn't threatened by this arrangement, she replies, "Of course I am. But at this point I think that asking Jenna to give up sex entirely would amount to a bigger threat than a few groupies. I can't imagine saying to her, 'Your body belongs to me whether I want it or not.'" Conscious that the juices of eros no longer flow between them, Arlene remakes the idea of fidelity. Monogamy stipulates keeping the forbidden on the outside, but rarely includes provisions for the couple. Eventually, if desire withers, monogamy too easily slides downward into celibacy. When this happens, fidelity becomes a weakness rather than a virtue.

In the twenty-five years that Marguerite and Ian have been together, they've had periods of total exclusivity and episodes of hurtful infidelity. "When I found out about Marguerite's affair I was devastated," Ian explains. "It took me months to realize I was also jealous. Not of her lover, but of her. Here I'd been resisting other women for years. When she came clean, we took stock. We decided to stay together but open the gates." Marguerite adds, "We're trying to come up with something that works for us. It isn't meant to be a recipe for others." When I ask her if her open marriage isn't painful, she answers, "Sometimes it is. Sometimes it's not. But monogamy—which we never negotiated, by the way—was painful, too."

Skeptics scoff at these arrangements, and question the level of commitment in these relationships. "I've never seen an open marriage last." "Try it for a while, then get back to me." "It's selfish." "Self-indulgent." "When you play with fire someone always gets burned."

Yet it's been my experience that couples who negotiate sexual boundaries, like the ones mentioned above, are no less committed than those who keep the gates closed. In fact, it is their desire to make the relationship stronger that leads them to explore other models of long-term love. Rather than expelling the third from the province of matrimony, they grant it a tourist visa.

For these couples, fidelity is defined not by sexual exclusivity but by the strength of their commitment. The boundaries aren't physical but emotional. The primacy of the couple remains paramount. The couples stress emotional monogamy as a sine qua non, and from there they make all sorts of sexual allowances. But far from being a hedonistic free-for-all, these relationships have explicit contracts which are renegotiated periodically, as the need arises. Marguerite and Ian emphasize that their arrangement is both clear and flexible. "We have our rules—no ongoing affairs, no lovers in the city where we live, no affairs with mutual friends—and as long as we stick to them things seem to be OK. If we need to renegotiate later, we'll do that."

It's interesting to note that although these couples bring a new meaning to the concept of fidelity, they are nonetheless susceptible to betrayal. Trust is crucial in any relationship, and this is no different for those who invite the third into their intimate space. Infidelity lies in breaches of the agreement, in violations of trust. Even though the rules themselves may look very different, they are breakable, and breaking them has equally painful consequences. In this sense, sexually open couples are no different from their monogamous counterparts.

Faced with the complications of affairs, divorce, and remarriage, some of my patients attempt a different course. Nonmonogamous people value the freedom of sexual expression, and they try to reconcile the perennials of love with the surprises of desire, hoping to resist the lassitude that creeps in with time. To repeat Marguerite's words, this is not a recipe for everyone.

The presence of the third is a fact of life; how we deal with it is up to us. We can approach it with fear, avoidance, and moral outrage; or we can bring to it a robust curiosity and a sense of intrigue. In his steamy affair, Doug courts it secretly. Bill's devastation is born of a desperate attempt to deny it. Selena and Max invite it in fantasy, but draw the line there. Joan and Hiro escort the third straight into their bedroom.

Marriage has become a matter of love; love is a matter of choice; and choice implies renouncing others. But that doesn't mean the others are dead. Nor does it mean that we need to deaden our senses so as to protect ourselves from their allure.

Acknowledging the third has to do with validating the erotic separateness of our partner. It follows that our partner's sexuality does not belong to us. It isn't just for and about us, and we should not assume that it rightfully falls within our jurisdiction. It doesn't. Perhaps that is true in action, but certainly not in thought. The more we choke each other's freedom, the harder it is for desire to breathe within a committed relationship.

Pursue the logic, and you have the itinerary for an emotionally enlarging journey. It goes something like this: I know you look at others, but I can't fully know what you see. I know others are looking at you, but I don't really know who it is they're seeing. Suddenly you're no longer familiar. You're no longer a known entity that I need not bother being curious about. In fact, you're quite a mystery. And I'm a little unnerved. Who are you? I want you.

Accommodating the third opens up an erotic expanse where eros needn't worry about wilting. In that expanse, we can be deeply moved by our partner's otherness, and soon thereafter deeply aroused.

I'd like to suggest that we view monogamy not as a given but as a choice. As such, it becomes a negotiated decision. More to the point, if we're planning to spend fifty years with one soul—and we want a happy jubilee—it may be wiser to review our contract at various junctures. Just how accommodating each couple may be to the third varies. But at least a nod is more apt to sustain desire with our one and only over the long haul—and perhaps even to create a new "art of loving" for the twenty-first century couple.

11

Putting the X Back in Sex
Bringing the Erotic Home

Love never dies a natural death. It dies because we don't know how to replenish its source.

—Anaïs Nin

It takes courage to push yourself to places that you have never been before . . . to test your limits . . . to break through barriers. And the day came when the risk it took to remain tight inside the bud was more painful than the risk it took to blossom.

—Anaïs Nin

IT ALWAYS AMAZES ME HOW much people are willing to experiment sexually outside their relationships, yet how tame and puritanical they are at home with their partners. Many of my patients have, by their own account, domestic lives devoid of excitement and eroticism, yet they are consumed and aroused by a richly imaginative sexual life beyond domesticity—affairs, pornography, cybersex, feverish daydreams. For them, sexual love becomes compromised in the making of a family, even a family of two. They numb themselves erotically. Then, having denied themselves freedom, and freedom of imagination, in their relationships, they go outside to reimagine themselves liberated from the constraints of commitment. Security inside, adventure and passion outside. So when the media frantically (yet regularly) announce that couples are not having sex, I can't help thinking that they may be having plenty of sex, but not with each other.

Passion may fuel the initial stages of a relationship, or it may not. Either way, the volatility of passionate eroticism is expected to evolve into a more staid, stable, and manageable alternative: mature love. Even the biochemistry of passion is known to be short-lived. The evolutionary anthropologist Helen Fisher says that the hormonal cocktail of romance (dopamine, norepineprine, and PEA) is known to last no more than a few years at best. Oxytocin, the cuddling hormone, outlasts them all. The fruits of this ripening love—companionship, deep respect, mutuality, and care—are considered by many to be a fair trade for erotic heat. If attraction and desire were the central actors in your courtship, now they retreat backstage to make way for the main act: building a life together.

Eroticism is conspicuously absent from our idea of marriage. Of course, committed couples are expected to have sex, and even to enjoy it these days. Sex solely for the sake of reproduction is, theoretically, passé. But sex and eroticism are not the same, and the lascivious, intimate, ardent, needful, frivolous, erotic sex of lovers becomes rare after the housewarming party. In spite of the sexually saturated media that promise unfettered excitement provided we follow the ten ideas suggested in this week's issue, there is still some anti-hedonism surrounding domesticated sex. Could it be that we're inundated with articles about how to make sex hot with our partners because we don't actually believe it can be hot with our partners? More to the point, could we believe deep down that it's not supposed to be? Could we believe that regardless of how sexually free we might have been before tying the knot, marriage is no place for the naughtiness of lust?

If marriage is about love, as we like to believe, then married sex must be a declaration of love. It has to be meaningful. But, the sex therapist Dagmar O'Connor says:

> For [married] sex to be "meaningful," it must always be an expression of love—preferably of lifelong, abiding love—every time we climb into bed with one another. And what an incredible burden that is! It eliminates sex stimulated by a whole array of other emotions and sensations: playful sex and angry sex, quick, "mindless" sex and "naughty" sex. It eliminates, in fact, just about every occasion for having sex there is. After all, who can feel "lifelong, abiding love" that regularly—especially at eleven o'clock at night?

Marriage, we've been taught, is about commitment, security, comfort, and family. It's a serious business, a responsible and purposeful enterprise; it's all the things we need, and all the things we need to do. Play and its playmates (risk, seduction, naughtiness, transgression) are left to fend for themselves outside the solid architecture of our homes.

Many people in my field assume that the intensity that shapes the early stages of romance is a sort of temporary insanity, destined to be cured by the rigors of the long haul. Clinicians often interpret the lust for sexual adventure—ranging from simple flirting to infatuation, from maintaining contact with previous lovers to cross-dressing, threesomes, and fetishes—as an infantile fantasy or a fear of commitment. They favor a model of love as a companionate, intimate, collaborative partnership. What we are left with is a relationship that is strong on cooperation and communication but weak on complicity and playfulness. But dispassionate friendship is a problematic ecology for cultivating eroticism.

The Day I Got That Ring . . .

Jacqueline and Philip are trying to rekindle the spark they once had. Married for ten years, they are finally emerging from the haze of parenting young children. This fall their youngest son began kindergarten, and his new schedule put some order back into theirs. At the same time, in the past year their friends have gone through an epidemic of divorces. "All these couples we used to hang out with, who got married right around the same time as us, are throwing in the towel," Philip tells me. "It makes you think about what you value, and it puts you face to face with the fatal flaws in your own relationship."

"And your fatal flaw?" I ask them.

"Sex," he answers.

"Cheating," she says.

When they met, Jacqueline was the winning prize for Philip. "Jackie was smart, beautiful, and sexy. I couldn't believe she was interested in me. I was really into her. I was all over her, too. We had great sex for a long time. Right up until I asked her to marry me," he recalls.

"What happened when she said yes?" I inquire.

"Nothing happened, but something did change when I got that ring. I didn't make the connection at the time, but now I see it pretty clearly. Entering a family shut me down fast. I didn't tell her about it. In fact, I even tried to deny to myself that anything was different. But pretty soon, I couldn't get turned on by her. Eventually, every time she left town, or even if she was just out for the night, I was logging on or trolling the bars."

Eight years of transgressions followed, some discovered, some disclosed, some mercifully kept secret. The sequence became repetitive, the resolution of one episode led to the next wave of transgression. Philip's shame at cheating was always followed by remorse and repentance. He felt terrible about hurting Jackie, and vowed to change. He would make a big show of being an upstanding man and a good husband, and she would forgive him and take him back. Then he would become restless, and a lecherous escalation would always follow. During these years they also had two sons, Jackie finished her first novel, Philip got tenure at a university, and they moved to New York. All these developments helped them put off dealing with the problem. But the latest round was, for Jackie, one too many.

To understand Philip's sexuality, I followed the link to his parents, whose marriage strikingly represented the cultural division between "safe" domesticity and "dangerous" eroticism. While his mother raised five kids, his father engaged in a continuous series of affairs, none of which he made great efforts to hide. Philip's grandfather, as it turns out, had done the same. "My father, who was actually a very likable man, went about it without much regard for how it made the rest of us feel—least of all my mom," Philip told me. His mother, whose suffering was severe, was nonetheless a practical woman who never forgot that she had five kids to feed. "She never spoke about it, but we all knew she needed us as much as we needed her."

In order not to upset her any further, Philip tried to be as different from his father as possible. He became what he calls an asexual wunderkind. "I was intensely moralistic and judgmental," Philip said ruefully. "On the surface I was the nice, safe guy girls went out with because they knew they could trust me not to take advantage of them; but underneath I was all over the place, and I hated myself for it." As an adolescent, Philip developed a compelling secret taste for pornography. When he became older, and actual sex became an option, he looked for women he could pick up on the fly for brief, inconsequential one-night stands. "Somehow, those rigid morals just fueled my obsession to break the rules." For Philip, defiance of ordinary decency was the key to his inner system of arousal. Sex, objectification, and transgression became one. Ironically, by segregating his sexuality outside the boundaries of his relationship with Jackie, Phillip hopes to protect her from the dangers of his desire.

Needless to say, Jackie was very disturbed by the loss of intensity in their sex life. Never very confident about her own magnetism, she, too, had been amazed by Philip's attraction to her. When it dwindled, she assumed he'd simply lost interest, and that this was to be expected. Growing up with a brother who was in and out of psychiatric institutions, she was accustomed to keeping her own needs to a minimum. She had learned not to impose herself and instead to take what she could get.

While Philip seeks affirmation on the outside, Jackie's self-affirmation rests solely on him and his response to her. She highlights a common way women order their sexuality, in that she makes him, and his desire for her, the centerpiece of her sexual identity. In the early days, when Philip was all over her, she blossomed. There was no issue. She felt open, daring, sexy, and wanted. Today, a good student of her own childhood, she avoids putting herself out there for fear of rejection. When she does get up the courage to make advances, Philip feels pressure to be responsive and to take care of her. "Whenever Jackie comes on to me, I'm paralyzed," he confides. "Which heightens Jackie's insecurity," I add.

Arguably, male desire runs the gamut between two extremes: those who plead for their partner to come on to them, thereby confirming their desirability; and those who balk when their mate initiates, fearful that their passivity isn't adequately masculine. Forever unsure of their power as Mom's little ward, the come-on averse walk a fine line between boyhood and manhood. Predictably, Philip takes Jackie's overtures as needy demands rather than tempting invitations.

Philip feels guilty because he can't be more erotically involved with his wife. When I ask him for a sexual image that includes her, he conjures up a picture of the two of them kissing romantically in the sunset. He adds that he has difficulty, now, imagining Jackie in a passionate, erotic way. He tells her openly, "I just can't see you in my mind as a sexual woman, and I feel bad about it, but it's the truth." Philip yearns for ardor with Jackie, but he believes that the tug-of-war within himself won't allow it. He dreads the rough edge of his desire within the bonds of holy matrimony, and is embarrassed by his need for objectified sex. To his thinking, love is no place for these wanton inclinations.

"You Don't Do That with Your Wife"

Many of my patients are afraid to express their intense sexual excitement with the one they love and respect. Philip is not alone in hiding his lack of desire behind the decency alibi. You may recognize some of these comments: "I can't imagine him saying what I want to hear. He'd wonder what happened to his wife." "I don't even want to think about, let alone talk about, what I was into before we met." "I can't do that with my wife." Domestic eroticism is wrapped in a veil of appropriateness.

When Philip tells me that Jackie would never go for this stuff, I ask him, "And the stuff is what exactly?" I am prepared for a long list of hard-core kink, and I am surprised when he reveals the basic menu of his sexual imagination. "I'm not one for subtleties. I like the blatant stuff. I like toys, lingerie, porn, a lot of graphic talk. Straightforward, honest fucking."

"All of which you and Jackie enjoyed before the ring?" I ask.

"Yeah." He shrugs.

"And now Jackie won't go for it? Or you won't go for it with her? I don't get a sense that she's changed all that much. But I wonder to what extent you feel that this is not stuff you do with your wife. You seem to believe that it's wrong to objectify someone you love."

"Are you saying it's not?" he asks.

"I'm saying it doesn't have to be. You know, a lot of couples play with objectification as a way to superimpose otherness on a partner who's become too familiar. It is often dismissed as lacking intimacy, but I think that when both of you are into it, it's another kind of closeness. You have to trust people a lot to let yourself forget them."

We segregate lust for psychological as well as cultural reasons. Any experience of love holds within it a dimension of dependence. In fact, dependence is an essential ingredient of connection. But it's a producer of terrific anxiety, because it implies that the one we love wields power over us. This is the power to love us, but also to abandon us. Fear—of judgment, of rejection, of loss—is embedded in romantic love. Sexual rejection at the hands of the one we love is particularly hurtful. We are therefore less inclined to be erotically adventurous with the person we depend on for so much and whose opinion is paramount. We'd rather edit ourselves, maintaining a tightly negotiated, acceptable, even boring erotic script, than risk injury. It is no surprise that some of us can freely engage in the perils and adventures of sex only when the emotional stakes are lower—when we love less or, more important, when we are less afraid to lose love. Stephen Mitchell writes, "It is not that romance necessarily fades over time, but it does become riskier."

Jackie has been listening attentively, and is patiently awaiting her turn. "I hear all this talk about edginess," she begins, "but with me he's almost giddy, more like a twelve-year-old boy than a man. It's hard to really unleash my sexuality with an adolescent. Why does he think he has to go out for this? Maybe I should buy a wig and belly up to the bar," she jokes.

"Not a bad idea," I answer.

I-Chat with Your Spouse

I point out that the way Philip has compartmentalized his sexuality, with loving sex at home and hot sex reserved for strangers, has banned eroticism from their relationship. Their repertoire is limited. But he isn't the only one at fault. For her part, Jackie has transferred her sense of sexual self-worth to him, and I recommend that she take it back. He should not have a monopoly on her sexuality. "Jackie, how long has it been since you flirted?" I ask her. "Can you open yourself up to the eyes of other men, so that Philip isn't the sole source of your sexual validation?" Philip starts to twitch in his chair.

"Just a minute," he says.

"Don't worry, I'm not suggesting tit for tat here," I reassure him. "But your wife is a very attractive woman, and if you can't see that, why shouldn't she hear it from someone else?"

Along these same lines, I also suggest that they create new E-mail accounts reserved exclusively for erotic exchanges between them—their thoughts, memories, fantasies, and seductions. I point out that this correspondence is not meant to be about the problems in their relationship, it is meant to be a space for play. I want them to use cyberspace to elicit curiosity, a sense of intrigue, and a kind of wholesome anxiety. Writing has many advantages over talking. You get to say your fill, craft your response, and give voice in writing to things your lips dare not utter. It provides a built-in distance, and I hope this will help dismantle their inhibitions.

By Valentine's Day Jackie has eased into the art of seduction. She's playful and daring, not only in her E-mails with Philip, but with other men as well. Several months later she tells me, "Your urging me to get a sense of myself from other men besides Philip has been very good for me." She started doing things with her male friends, going to concerts and galleries, and she has generally been more flirtatious. "Nothing big, you know, but it's been fun to be out there again, talking to men who are not my husband, knowing they enjoy my company. And now, Philip's every word or look isn't the most important thing in my life."

Jackie's new confidence has left Philip slightly unmoored, and that turns out to be a good thing. He is intrigued by the way she writes to him, and is surprised to find that in the graphic lexicon of sex, she can certainly hold her own. All this sexualizes her in his eyes. Freed from the predictability of a script, he takes a second look. The pseudo anonymity of their E-mails has allowed him to see her as a subject with her own desires, turning her into the object of his desire. "I'm saying things to her that I never thought I could. I expected she'd be turned off, but she's not. She needs a lot less taking care of than I projected onto her," Philip admits. "I realized I put a lot of stuff on her that doesn't belong to her. It belongs to me, or at least to my family."

"I don't get how your flings were supposed to be taking care of me, though I know in your mind it makes sense," Jackie tells him. "It's not OK, but I understand it. Still, I was always surprised at how easily you let yourself be caught. Like you were asking for it, so you could come to Mommy and get punished. I'm not interested in replaying your family drama. I'll leave you first, and you know it." To me she says, "Realizing I had the strength to leave helped me make the choice to stay. I have a lot more freedom. When I initiate sex now, I can feel almost brazen, and I like that. 'You want this, Philip? Take it!' It doesn't have to be romantic or even particularly personal. I like a lot of different things. I prefer tender love, but sometimes greedy is good, too."

I've worked with Jackie and Philip on and off for years. Philip has stopped acting out, and over time he has searched for ways to undo the deeply ingrained belief that hot sex can't happen at home. By finding ways to experience himself as a sexual man who is also a faithful man, he was able to undo family patterns that were at least three generations old. In the past, Philip's fascination with porn was a haven for him, a fantasy of immediacy where the moment of desire and satisfaction merged. The women on the screen offered no resistance and required no effort on his part. Hence the tension between wanting and getting was nullified, and Philip never had to reconcile desire in the context of love. Gradually, he has allowed the dislocated parts of his sexuality to come home, and has been more able to remain present with his wife.

The ongoing challenge for Jackie and Philip is to continue to bring the erotic home—to experience small transgressions, illicit striving, and passionate idealization in the midst of their intimate lives. The English analyst Adam Phillips underscores this point in his book *Monogamy*:

> *If it is the forbidden that is exciting—if desire is fundamentally transgressive—then the monogamous are like the very rich. They have to find their poverty. They have to starve themselves enough. In other words they have to work, if only to keep what is always too available sufficiently illicit to be interesting.*

Can You Want What You Have?

Oscar Wilde wrote, "In this world there are only two tragedies. One is getting what one wants, and the other is not getting it." When our desires are unfulfilled, we are disappointed. It's frustrating to be denied a raise, a college acceptance, an audition. When the object of our desire is a person, her rejection leaves us feeling lonely, unworthy, unloved, or—worse—unlovable. But fulfilled desire carries its own brand of loss. Getting what we want undermines the thrill of wanting it. The deliciousness of yearning, the elaborate strategies of pursuit, the charged fantasies, in short all the activity and energy that went into wanting give way to the foreclosure of having. Just think about the last thing you had to have until you owned it. Now that it's yours, you may enjoy it, you may love it, but do you still want it? Do you even remember how much you wanted it in the first place? Gail Godwin wrote, "The act of longing will always be more intense than the requiting of it."

Is it harder to want what you already have? The law of diminishing returns tells us that increased frequency leads to decreased satisfaction. The more you use a product, the less satisfying each subsequent use will be. Paris just isn't the same on your fifteenth trip as it was on the first. Fortunately, the logic of this argument breaks down when it is applied to love, for it is based on the erroneous assumption that we can own a person in the same way that we can own an iPod or a new pair of Prada heels. When my friend Jane said, "Perhaps I only want what I can't have," I responded, "What makes you think you have your husband?"

The grand illusion of committed love is that we think our partners are ours. In truth, their separateness is unassailable, and their mystery is forever ungraspable. As soon as we can begin to acknowledge this, sustained desire becomes a real possibility. It's remarkable to me how a sudden threat to the status quo (an affair, an infatuation, a prolonged absence, or even a really good fight) can suddenly ignite desire. There's nothing like the fear of loss to make those old shoes look new again.

The counterargument to the law of diminishing returns is the principle that consistent investment leads to increased satisfaction. The more you do something, and the better you get at it, the more you're going to enjoy it. The weekly tennis player who continues to improve his game would argue for the positive effects of frequency. For her, Paris just keeps getting better. The more she practices, the stronger her skills. The stronger her skills, the deeper her confidence. The more confident she feels, the more risks she takes. The more risks she takes, the more exciting the game. Of course, all this practice takes effort and discipline. It is not just a matter of being in the mood; it requires patience and sustained attention. The tennis player knows intuitively that growth is rarely linear; she may experience some plateaus and some slowdowns, but the reward is worth the effort.

Unfortunately, all too often we associate effort with work, and discipline with pain. But there's a different way to think of work. It can be creative and life-affirming, sparking a heightened sense of vitality rather than a bone-deep exhaustion. If we want sex to be fulfilling, then we have to apply effort in just this artful way.

The Myth of Spontaneity

There is a powerful ideal operating in many people's view of sex— that it's an instant fit, a hand-in-pocket, skin-to-skin compatibility that is perfect from the start. Good sex is supposed to be easy, tension-free, and uninhibited. Either you have it or you don't. This idea is often accompanied by its good neighbor, the myth of spontaneity. The word "spontaneity" comes up like a mantra whenever men and women in my office talk about what constitutes, for them, exciting, thrilling, can't-wait, truly erotic sex. It is hard to overstate their enthusiastic conviction that really sexy sex is supposed to be spur-of-the-moment.

We like to believe that sex arises from an impulse or inclination that is natural, unprompted, and artless. We talk about being swept away. "I couldn't resist . . . I felt such a rush through my veins . . . It was bigger than both of us . . . I was completely taken over." This infatuation with the big bang theory of sex suggests our impatience with seduction and playful eroticism, which take up too much time, require too much effort, and—most important—demand full consciousness of what we are doing. For many of us, premeditated sex is suspicious. It threatens our belief that sex is subject only to the machinations of magic and chemistry. The idea that sex must be spontaneous keeps us one step removed from having to will sex, to own our desire, and to express it with intent. As long as sex is something that just happens, you don't have to claim it. It's ironic that in such a willful society, willfully conjuring up sex seems obvious and crass. It embarrasses us, as if we've been caught doing something inappropriate.

When my patients wax nostalgic about the early days of rapid-ignition sex, I remind them that even in the beginning, spontaneity was a myth. Whatever used to happen "in the moment" was often the result of hours, if not days, of preparation. What outfit, what conversation, which restaurant, which music? All that planning—that highly detailed, imaginative production—was part of the buildup and part of the denouement.

For this reason, I urge my patients not to be spontaneous about sex. Spontaneity is a fabulous idea, but in an ongoing relationship whatever is going to "just happen" already has. Now they have to make it happen. Committed sex is intentional sex. "I couldn't resist" has to become "I don't want to resist." "We just fell into each other's arms" has to become "Let me take you in my arms." "We just click" has to become "Can we click tonight?" My aim is to help patients become comfortable with sexuality as a consciously acknowledged and enthusiastically welcomed part of their lives—something that demands full engagement.

The idea of planning is a hurdle many couples need to cross. They associate planning with scheduling, scheduling with work, and work with obligation. Often, therapy is a process of dismantling these beliefs.

Bringing Intentionality to Sex

Dominick and Raoul complain about their lackluster sex life. In the early days of their romance, when Raoul still lived in Miami, distance precluded routine. Their weekends were much anticipated and never dull. But now, living together, they spend their downtime doing housework and running errands. I can't help noticing the discrepancy between the attention they devote to these chores and the lack of attention they bring to their sex life—as if sex operates according to a different principle.

"The laundry won't just do itself, you know," Dominick says defensively.

"And sex will?" I ask.

Dominick pretends not to understand what I mean by planned sex. "You want me to put it in my BlackBerry? Thursday night, ten o'clock? That seems so pathetic," he says.

"If you don't want sex to be another item on your to-do list, don't treat it like one," I respond. "I'm not talking about scheduling sex, I'm talking about creating an erotic space, and that takes time. What will occur in that space is open-ended, but the space itself is marked by intentionality. Like that osso buco you made for Raoul last weekend—it didn't just happen."

Dominick is a gourmet. On Saturday, he cooked Raoul a classic Italian stew. It started as a thought—that he'd like to do something nice. He played around with various ideas until he settled on the veal. Then he went to Little Italy for the finest meat, to a bakery in the Village for his favorite semolina bread, and to a specialty shop in SoHo for the chocolate cannoli. Finally, he schlepped all the way uptown for the perfect bottle of Montepulciano. The meal took most of the day, but in the end it was an epicurean delight, even an erotic experience. It was all planned for pleasure.

"Yeah, it's a lot of work," Dominick admits, "but I enjoy it, so it doesn't feel like drudgery."

"How is it that sex has come to feel like work to you? You seem reluctant to bring the same intent to your erotic life that you do to your cooking," I point out.

"It seems so contrived when it comes to sex," Dominick says.

Like Dominick and Raoul, quite a few of my patients balk at the idea of deliberateness when it comes to sex. They find these strategies too laborious for the long haul, believing they should no longer be necessary after the initial conquest. "Seducing my partner? Do I still have to do that?" This reluctance is often a covert expression of an infantile wish to be loved just as we are, without any effort whatsoever on our part, because we're so special. It's the grandiosity of the baby, and we all carry it inside. "I don't want to! Why should I? You're supposed to love me no matter what!" The sex therapist Margaret Nichols observes that though your partner may still love you if you gain fifty pounds and shuffle around the house in bunny slippers and a stained T-shirt, he probably won't get hard for you (and she won't get wet).

"Is the titillation of seduction only the privilege of those who date?" I ask Dominick. "Just because you live with someone doesn't necessarily mean he's readily available. If anything, he requires more attention, not less. If you want sex to remain humid, this is the kind of attention you have to bring to it. No, not every day, but once in a while can you make a meal of Raoul?"

Planning Creates Anticipation

Anticipation implies that we are looking forward to something. It is an important ingredient of desire, and planning for sex helps to generate it. When Dominick prepares his osso buco, he can almost taste it in advance. He imagines Raoul's surprise and pleasure. He hopes it will make his boyfriend feel special, and he envisions Raoul's gratitude. Fantasy is the mortar of anticipation. It's a way of imagining what something is going to be like. It's a kind of foreplay that takes place outside the couple's direct interaction. Anticipation is part of building a plot; that is why romance novels and soap operas are filled with it.

I believe that longing, waiting, and yearning are fundamental elements of desire that can be generated with forethought, even in long-term relationships. When Nile and Sarah go out on Saturday, they often have a few things planned. Dinner, music, and—later—sex. In the past, an entire evening's worth of wooing was undone the instant Sarah had to pay the babysitter. "All of a sudden, I'd be the mother again, and all that tension we worked to build up would just vanish. Now, Nile deals with the babysitter and I go straight to the bedroom. It's an arrangement that lets me keep up the momentum." Sarah and Nile have three kids who keep her running all day, every day. She has made it very clear to Nile that it takes a lot to get her out of that role, and very little for her to slip back in. "I used to think that it was a matter of being in the mood, but I was disabused of that idea a long time ago. Waiting for the mood is like waiting for the Second Coming. I like the planning. It gives me something to look forward to when I'm playing with Barbies and checking homework."

What Sarah looks forward to is more than the sex; it's the ritual. Spending ample time together, woman to man, they temporarily slip out of the chains of reality. Their foreplay lasts hours. They've been at this for twelve years, and like a mastered discipline, they miss it when they skip it. They know that great sex generally demands more than fifteen minutes right after the eleven o'clock news.

Cultivating Play

When couples complain that their sex life is listless, I know it isn't mere frequency they're after. They may want more, but they certainly want better. For this reason, I prefer to talk about their erotic life rather than about their sex life. The physical act of sex is too narrow a subject, which easily degenerates into a conversation about numbers. Human nature abhors a vacuum of intensity. People long for radiance. They want to feel alive. If given half a chance, loving partners can fill the intensity void with transcendence.

Animals have sex; eroticism is exclusively human. It is sexuality transformed by the imagination. In fact, you don't even need the act of sex to have a full erotic experience, though sex is often hinted at, envisioned. Eroticism is the cultivation of excitement, a purposeful quest for pleasure. Octavio Paz likens eroticism to the poetry of the body, the testimony of the senses. Like a poem, it is not linear; it meanders and twists back on itself. It shows us what we see not with our eyes but with the eyes of our spirit. Eroticism reveals to us another world inside this world. The senses become servants of the imagination, letting us see the invisible and hear the inaudible.

Eroticism, intertwined as it is with imagination, is another form of play. I think of play as an alternative reality midway between the actual and the fictitious, a safe space where we experiment, reinvent ourselves, and take chances. Through play we suspend disbelief—we pretend something is real even when we damn well know it is not. Earnestness has no place here.

Play, by definition, is carefree and unself-conscious. The great theoretician of play, Johan Huizinga, maintained that a fundamental feature of play is that it serves no other purpose. The purposelessness associated with play is hard to reconcile with our culture of high efficiency and constant accountability. More and more, we measure play by its benefits. We play squash for cardiovascular conditioning; we take our kids to dinner to expand their palates; we go on vacation to recharge. Yet if we're plagued by self-awareness, obsessed with outcomes, or fearful of judgment, our enjoyment is inevitably compromised.

When we are children, play comes to us naturally, but our capacity for play collapses as we age. Sex often remains the last arena of play we can permit ourselves, a bridge to our childhood. Long after the mind has been filled with injunctions to be serious, the body remains a free zone, unencumbered by reason and judgment. In lovemaking, we can recapture the utterly uninhibited movement of the child, who has not yet developed self-consciousness before the judging gaze of others.

Erotic Intelligence

Every so often, I meet couples who get it, who maintain a sense of playfulness with each other, in and out of the bedroom. They are physically and sensually alive—two people whose desire for one another hasn't been left to languish. Even in our culture of immediate gratification, they're able to see seduction as an end in itself. Johanna continues to bewitch her boyfriend of ten years by setting up rendezvous in motels in a nearby suburb. Darnell and his lover pretend not to know each other when they go to a party. Eric describes making love to his wife in the alley of their apartment building when they come home late at night, a furtive pleasure they indulge in before checking on the kids. Every year, Ivan and Rachel go away for a long weekend of consensual adultery with other swingers. "Instead of having secrets from each other, we have secrets from the world." Jessica has rescued her husband from many lonesome stretches on the road by teasing him on the CB radio. Every morning, Leo tells his wife how lucky he is to be married to her, and he still means it after more than fifty years.

For all these couples, playfulness is central to their relationship, and eroticism extends beyond the sexual act. Their lovemaking can be ceremonious or sudden, soulful or utilitarian, vanilla or transgressive, warm or hot. The point is that sex is pleasurable and inviting, not dutiful. They revere the erotic, yet they delight in its irreverence. They like sex, they especially like it with each other, and they take the time to nurture an erotic space.

Like all couples, they go through periods when desire is dormant—when they are estranged from each other, or simply immersed in their own projects and in their own lives—but they don't panic, terrified that something is fundamentally wrong with them. They know that erotic intensity waxes and wanes, that desire suffers periodic eclipses and intermittent disappearances. But given sufficient attention, they can bring the frisson back.

For them, love is a vessel that contains both security and adventure, and commitment offers one of the great luxuries of life: time. Marriage is not the end of their romance, it's the beginning. They know that they have years in which to deepen their connection, to experiment, to regress, and even to fail. They see their relationship as something alive and ongoing, not a fait accompli. It's a story that they are writing together, one with many chapters, and neither partner knows how it will end. There's always a place they haven't gone yet, always something about the other still to be discovered.

Modern relationships are cauldrons of contradictory longings: safety and excitement, grounding and transcendence, the comfort of love and the heat of passion. We want it all, and we want it with one person. Reconciling the domestic and the erotic is a delicate balancing act that we achieve intermittently at best. It requires knowing your partner while recognizing his persistent mystery; creating security while remaining open to the unknown; cultivating intimacy that respects privacy. Separateness and togetherness alternate, or proceed in counterpoint. Desire resists confinement, and commitment mustn't swallow freedom whole.

At the same time, eroticism in the home requires active engagement and willful intent. It is an ongoing resistance to the message that marriage is serious, more work than play; and that passion is for teenagers and the immature. We must unpack our ambivalence about pleasure, and challenge our pervasive discomfort with sexuality, particularly in the context of family. Complaining of sexual boredom is easy and conventional. Nurturing eroticism in the home is an act of open defiance.

Notes

1: From Adventure to Captivity

1 The original primordial fire: Octavio Paz. 1995. *The Double Flame: Love and Eroticism*. San Diego, Calif.: Harvest, p. x.

3 Hence the division between the romantics and the realists: Ethel Spector Person. 1988. *Dreams of Love and Fateful Encounters: The Power of Romantic Passion*. New York: Penguin.

4 Stephen Mitchell: Stephen A. Mitchell. 2002. *Can Love Last?: The Fate of Romance over Time*. New York: Norton.

8 Anthony Giddens describes: Anthony Giddens. 1992. *The Transformation of Intimacy: Sexuality, Love and Eroticism in Modern Societies*. Stanford, Calif.: Stanford University Press.

10 The motivational expert Anthony Robbins: At a workshop in Fiji, 2005.

11 As Stephen Mitchell points out: *Can Love Last?*, p. 44.

11 In the words of Proust: Marcel Proust, from http://www.quotation spage.com/quote/31288.html.

18 Mark Epstein explains: Mark Epstein. 2005. *Open to Desire: Embracing a Lust for Life*. New York: Gotham, p. 45.

2: More Intimacy, Less Sex

19   Love and lust: Jack Morin. 1995. *The Erotic Mind*. New York: Harper-Collins, p. 200.

20   Ethel Specter Person writes: Ethel Spector Person. 1988. *Dreams of Love and Fateful Encounters: The Power of Romantic Passion*. New York: W.W. Norton, p. 30.

23   Dr. Patricia Love gives voice: Patricia Love and Jo Robinson. 1995. *Hot Monogamy: Essential Steps to More Passionate, Intimate Lovemaking*. New York: Plume. p. 95.

25   The psychologist Michael Vincent Miller: Michael Vincent Miller. 1995. *Intimate Terrorism: The Crisis of Love in an Age of Disillusion*. New York: Norton, p. 39.

29   The psychoanalyst Michael Bader: Michael J. Bader. 2002. *Arousal: The Secret Logic of Sexual Fantasies*. New York: St. Martin's.

32   The sex therapist Dagmar O'Connor: Dagmar O'Connor. 1986. *How to Make Love to the Same Person for the Rest of Your Life and Still Love It*. London: Virgin.

36   The psychologist Virginia Goldner: Virginia Goldner. 2004. "Review Essay: Attachment and Eros—Opposed or Synergistic?" *Psa Dialogues*, 14(3), pp. 381–96.

36   Simone de Beauvoir writes: Simone de Beauvoir. 1952. *The Second Sex*. New York: Knopf, p. 446.

36   The French psychologist Jacques Salomé: Jacques Salomé. 2002. *Jamais seuls ensemble: Comment vivre à deux en restant différents*. Québec: Éditions de l'Homme, p. 13.

3: The Pitfalls of Modern Intimacy

38   We have no secrets: Carly Simon, from the album *No Secrets,* Elektra/Asylum Records, 1972.

39   Tevye, in *Fiddler on the Roof:* Joseph Stein. 2004. *Fiddler on the Roof: Based on the Sholom Aleichem Stories*. New York: Limelight. (Reprint of original script, Pocket Books, 1965.)

40   The family therapist Lyman Wynne: Lyman C. Wynne and A. R. Wynne. 1986. "The Quest for Intimacy." *Journal of Marital and Family Therapy,* 12, p. 389.

45   David Schnarch deftly illustrates: David Schnarch. 1991. *Passionate Marriage: Keeping Love and Intimacy Alive in Committed Relationships.* New York: Holt, p.107.

51   The family therapist Kaethe Weingarten: Kaethe Weingarten. 1991 "The Discourses of Intimacy: Adding a Social Constructionist and Feminist View," *Family Process,* 30, pp. 285–305.

4: Democracy Versus Hot Sex

53   No bill of sexual rights: Daphne Merkin. 2000. "The Last Taboo." *The New York Times,* December 3.

59   Mordechai Gafni, a scholar of Jewish mysticism: Mordechai Gafni. 2003. "On the Erotic and the Ethical." *Tikkun Magazine,* April–May.

62   Ethel Spector Person: Ethel Spector Person. 2002. *Feeling Strong: The Achievement of Authentic Power.* New York: Morrow, p. xi.

63   Stephen Mitchell makes the point: Stephen A. Mitchell. 2002. *Can Love Last? The Fate of Romance over Time.* New York: Norton, p.144.

69   They were primarily a practice of gay men: Anthony Giddens. 1992. *The Transformation of Intimacy: Sexuality, Love and Eroticism in Modern Societies.* Stanford, Calif.: Stanford University Press, p. 123.

69   The social critic Camille Paglia: From www.urbandesires.com issue 1.2 January–February 1995. Interview with Tracy Quan, "The Prostitute, the Comedian, and Me."

5: Can Do!

71   Energy and persistence: Benjamin Franklin, http://www.quotations page.com/quote/34574.html.

72   Laura Kipnis writes: Laura Kipnis. 2003. *Against Love: A Polemic.* New York: Pantheon, p. 67.

73   You break the problem down to its component parts: Ronald A. Heifetz. 1994. *Leadership without Easy Answers*. New York: Belknap, p. 69.

73   The sex therapist Leonore Tiefer: Leonore Tiefer. 1995. *Sex Is Not a Natural Act and Other Essays*. Boulder, Col.: Westview, p. 51.

73   *Newsweek* magazine: Kathleen Deveny. June 30, 2003, "We're Not in the Mood." *Newsweek*, p.41.

74   French author Jean-Claude Guillebaud: Jean-Claude Guillebaud. 1998. *La Tyrannie du plaisir*. Paris: Éditions du Seuil.

74   Medicine knows how to scare: Pascal Bruckner and Alain Finkielkraut. 1977. *Le Nouveau Désordre amoureux*. Paris: Éditions du Seuil.

74   The "sexual performance perfection industry": Barry A. Bass. 2001. "The Sexual Performance Perfection Industry and the Medicalization of Male Sexuality." *Family Journal: Counseling and Therapy for Couples and Families*, 9, pp. 337–40.

75   As Adam Phillips wryly notes: Adam Phillips. 1996. *Monogamy*. New York: Vintage, p. 62.

75   Octavio Paz writes: Octavio Paz. 1995. *The Double Flame: Love and Eroticism*. San Diego, Calif.: Harvest, p. 162.

76   We don't always know our aims in advance: Francesco Alberoni. 1987. *L'érotisme*. Paris: Éditions Ramsey, p. 136.

79   There's an evolutionary anthropologist named Helen Fisher: Helen Fisher. 2004. *Why We Love: The Nature and Chemistry of Romantic Love*. New York: Holt.

82   It belongs to the category of existential dilemmas: Barry Johnson. 1992. *Polarity Management: Identifying and Managing Unsolvable Problems*. Middleville, Mich.: Polarity Management Associates (PMA).

82   Barry Johnson, an expert on leadership: Ibid.

83   What Octavio Paz calls "a swamp of concupiscence": *The Double Flame*, p. 49.

87   I give him the following quotation from buddhist yoga teacher Frank Jude Boccio: www.judekaruna.net/yoga

6: Sex Is Dirty; Save It for Someone You Love

88   Sex without sin: Luis Buñuel, quoted in Daphne Merkin. 2000. "The Last Taboo." *New York Times*, December 3.

88   I regret to say: http://en.thinkexist.com/quotation/i_regret_to_say_that_we_of_the_fbi_are_powerless/7865.html.

90   Sex is everywhere, in all its permutations: Lillian Rubin. 1990. *Intimate Strangers: Men and Women Together*. New York: HarperPerennial, p. 9.

91   The blatant marketing of sexual images: Jean-Claude Guillebaud. 1998. *La Tyrannie du plaisir*. Paris: Éditions du Seuil.

92   It's also worth noting that in Europe: Linda Berne, Ed.D., and Barbara Huberman, M.Ed. "European Approaches to Adolescent Sexual Behavior and Responsibility: Executive Summary and Call to Action." Washington, DC: Advocates for Youth, 1999.

7: Erotic Blueprints

106   Grown-ups never understand: Antoine de Saint-Exupéry. 1943 *The Little Prince*, trans. by Richard Howard. New York: Harcourt.

106   So, like a forgotten fire: Gaston Bachelard, from http://en.thinkexist.com/quotation/so-like-a-forgotten-fire-a-childhood-can-always/363615.html.

109   The sex therapist Jack Morin: Jack Morin. 1995. *The Erotic Mind*. New York: HarperCollins, p. 115.

111   As Roland Barthes wrote: Roland Barthes. 1977. *Fragments d'un discours amoureux*. Paris: Éditions du Seuil, p. 44.

113   The psychoanalyst Jessica Benjamin writes: Jessica Benjamin. 1988. *The Bonds of Love: Psychoanalysis, Feminism, and the Problem of Domination*. New York: Pantheon, p. 98.

122   Michael Bader links the idea of selfishness: Michael J. Bader. 2002. *Arousal: The Secret Logic of Sexual Fantasies*. New York: St. Martin's, p. 147.

8: Parenthood

125   Anne Roiphe. 2002. *Married: A Fine Predicament.* New York: Basic Books, pp. 149–50.

132   The Italian historian Francesco Alberoni: Francesco Alberoni. 1987. L'érotisme. Paris: Éditions Ramsey, p. 28.

138   *Sexy Mamas,* by Cathy Winks and Anne Semans: Cathy Winks and Anne Semans. 2004. *Sexy Mamas: Keeping Your Sex Life Alive While Raising Kids.* New York: Inner Ocean Publishing.

145   Adam Gopnik contrasts America's asexual model of reproduction: Adam Gopnick. 2001. *Paris to the Moon.* New York: Random House, pp. 299, 301.

9: Of Flesh and Fantasy

152   The whole fauna of human fantasies: Louis Aragon, from http:// en.thinkexist.com/quotation/the_whole_fauna_of_human_fantasies-their_ marine/323656.html.

156   The psychoanalyst Michael Bader: Michael J. Bader. 2002. *Arousal: The Secret Logic of Sexual Fantasies.* New York: St. Martin's.

157   Nancy Friday writes: Nancy Friday. 1992. *The Erotic Impulse: Honoring the Sensual Self.* David Steinberg, ed. New York: Tarcher, p. 14.

167   The sex therapist Jack Morin: Jack Morin. 1995. *The Erotic Mind.* New York: HarperCollins, p. 101.

171   Heterosexual pornography, predominantly produced by and for men: Anthony Giddens. 1992. *The Transformation of Intimacy: Sexuality, Love and Eroticism in Modern Societies.* Stanford, Calif.: Stanford University Press, p. 119.

10: Monogamy

175   Are there any secrets: Alain de Botton. 1998. *How Proust Can Change Your Life.* New York: Vintage, p. 171.

175   The bonds of wedlock: Alexandre Dumas, from http://www.jimpoz. com/quotes/category.asp?categoryid=42.

177   The Brazilian family therapist Michele Scheinkman: Michele Scheinkman. 2005. "Beyond the Trauma of Betrayal: Reconsidering Affairs in Couples Therapy." *Family Process*, 44, pp. 227–44.

179   Hence the psychologist Erich Fromm makes the point: Erich Fromm. 1956. *The Art of Loving*. New York: Harper and Row, p. 43.

179   The feminist psychoanalyst Nancy Chodorow: Nancy Chodorow. 1978. *The Reproduction of Mothering: Psychoanalysis and the Sociology of Gender*. Berkeley: University of California Press, p. 194.

188   Adam Phillips writes: Adam Phillips. 1996. *Monogamy*. New York: Vintage.

189   Laura Kipnis says: Laura Kipnis. 2000. *Against Love: A Polemic*. New York: Pantheon, p. 78.

190   Excessive monitoring can set the stage: Stephen A. Mitchell. 2002. *Can Love Last? The Fate of Romance over Time*. New York: Norton, p. 51.

190   The psychologist Janet Reibstein: Janet Reibstein and Martin Richards. 1993. *Sexual Arrangements: Marriage and the Temptation of Infidelity*. New York: Scribner, p. 73.

195   Adam Philips makes the point: Adam Phillips. 1996. *Monogamy*. New York: Vintage, preface.

196   The anthropologist Katherine Frank wryly notes: "Play Couples in Paradise: Touristic Sexuality and Lifestyle Travel." Unpublished.

11: Putting the X Back in Sex

200   Love never dies a natural death: Anaïs Nin from http://en.thinkexist.com/quotes/anais_nin/

200   It takes courage: Ibid.

201   The evolutionary anthropologist Helen Fisher: Helen Fisher. "The Drive to Love." Keynote address at the "Challenging Couples, Challenging Therapists" conference, sponsored by the Milton H. Erikson Foundation, Los Angeles, CA, May 28, 2004.

202   The sex therapist Dagmar O'Connor says: Dagmar O'Connor. 1986.

How to Make Love to the Same Person for the Rest of Your Life and Still Love It. London: Virgin, p. 37.

207   **Stephan Mitchell writes:** Stephen A. Mitchell. 2002. *Can Love Last? The Fate of Romance over Time.* New York: Norton, p. 114.

210   **Adam Phillips underscores this point:** Adam Phillips. 1996. *Monogamy.* New York: Vintage, p. 11.

210   **Oscar Wilde wrote:** Oscar Wilde. 1892. *Lady Windermere's Fan,* Act III.

211   **Gail Godwin wrote:** Gail Godwin from http://en.thinkexist.com/quotation/the_act_of_longing_for_something_will_always_be/184996.html.

215   **The sex therapist Margaret Nichols:** Margaret Nichols. 1987. "What Feminists Can Learn from the Lesbian Sex Radicals." *Conditions: Fourteen,* ed. Conditions Collective. New York, pp. 152–63.

217   **Octavio Paz likens eroticism:** Octavio Paz. 1995. *The Double Flame: Love and Eroticism.* San Diego, Calif.: Harvest, p. 2.

217   **The great theoretician of play, Johan Huizinga:** *Homo Ludens.* 1971. Boston, Mass.: Beacon Press.

Bibliography

Books

Alberoni, Francesco. 1987. *L'érotisme*. Paris: Éditions Ramsay.

Alberoni, Francesco. 1983. *Falling in Love*. New York: Random House.

Angier, Natalie. 1999. *Woman: An Intimate Geography*. Boston, Mass.: Houghton Mifflin.

Bader, Michael J. 2002. *Arousal: The Secret Logic of Sexual Fantasies*. New York: St. Martin's.

Badinter, Elisabeth. 1992. *XY: De l'identité masculine*. Paris: Éditions Odile Jacob.

Baker, Mark. 1994. *Sex Lives: A Sexual Self-Portrait of America*. New York: Simon and Schuster.

Barthes, Roland. 1977. *Fragments d'un discours amoureux*. Paris: Éditions du Seuil.

Bataille, Georges. 1962. *Eroticism: Death and Sensuality*. New York: Walker. (Originally published 1957. Paris: Éditions de Minuit.)

Baudrillard, Jean. 1990. *Seduction*. New York: St. Martin's. (Originally published 1979. Paris: Éditions Galilée.)

Beck, Charlotte Joko. 1989. *Everyday Zen: Love and Work*. New York: HarperCollins.

Benjamin, Jessica. 1988. *The Bonds of Love: Psychoanalysis, Feminism, and the Problem of Domination*. New York: Pantheon.

Blumstein, Philip, and Pepper Schwartz, eds. 1983. *American Couples: Money, Work, Sex*. New York: Morrow.

Botton, Alain de. 1998. *How Proust Can Change Your Life*. New York: Vintage.

Boyarin, Daniel. 1993. *Carnal Israel: Reading Sex in Talmudic Culture*. Berkeley: University of California Press.

Brooks, Gary. 1995. *The Centerfold Syndrome: How Men Can Overcome Objectification and Achieve Intimacy with Women*. San Francisco, Calif.: Jossey-Bass.

Bruckner, Pascal, and Alain Finkielkraut. 1977. *Le Nouveau Désordre amoureux*. Paris: Éditions du Seuil.

Caplan, Pat, ed. 1987. *The Cultural Construction of Sexuality*. London: Tavistock.

Chedzogy, Kate, Melanie Hansen, and Suzanne Trill, eds. 1997. *Voicing Women: Gender and Sexuality in Early Modern Writing*. Pittsburgh, Pa.: Duquesne University Press.

Chodorow, Nancy. 1978. *The Reproduction of Mothering: Psychoanalysis and the Sociology of Gender*. Berkeley: University of California Press.

Davis, Michele Weiner. 2003. *The Sex-Starved Marriage: A Couple's Guide to Boosting Their Marriage Libido*. New York: Simon and Schuster.

de Beauvoir, Simone. 1952. *The Second Sex*. New York: Knopf.

De Marneffe, Daphne. 2004. *Maternal Desire: On Children, Love, and the Inner Life*. Boston, Mass.: Little, Brown.

Epstein, Mark. 2005. *Open to Desire: Embracing a Lust for Life*. New York: Gotham.

Fillion, Kate. 1996. *Lip Service: The Truth about Women's Darker Side in Love, Sex, and Friendship*. New York: HarperCollins.

Fisher, Helen. 2004. *Why We Love: The Nature and Chemistry of Romantic Love*. New York: Holt.

Frank, Katherine. 2002. *G-Strings and Sympathy: Strip Club Regulars and Male Desire*. Durham, N.C.: Duke University Press.

Friday, Nancy. 1992. *The Erotic Impulse: Honoring the Sensual Self*. David Steinberg, ed. New York: Tacher.

Friday, Nancy. 1991. *Women on Top: How Real Life Has Changed Women's Sexual Fantasies*. New York: Simon and Schuster.

Fromm, Erich. 1956. *The Art of Loving*. New York: Harper and Row.

Giddens, Anthony. 1992. *The Transformation of Intimacy: Sexuality, Love, and Eroticism in Modern Societies*. Stanford, Calif.: Stanford University Press.

Gopnick, Adam. 2001. *Paris to the Moon*. New York: Random House.

Gilbert, Harriett. 1993. *Fetishes, Florentine Girdles, and Other Explorations into the Sexual Imagination*. New York: HarperPerennial.

Gottman, John. 1994. *Why Marriages Succeed or Fail . . . and How You Can Make Yours Last*. New York: Simon and Schuster.

Guillebaud, Jean-Claude. 1998. *La Tyrannie du plaisir*. Paris: Éditions du Seuil.

Hanauer, Cathi, ed. 2003. *The Bitch in the House: 26 Women Tell the Truth about Sex, Solitude, Work, Motherhood, and Marriage*. New York: HarperPerennial, Reprint Edition.

Heifetz, Ronald A. 1994. *Leadership without Easy Answers*. New York: Belknap.

Heyn, Dalma. 1992. *The Erotic Silence of the American Wife*. New York: Plume.

Illouz, Eva. 1997. *Consuming the Romantic Utopia: Love and the Cultural Contradictions of Capitalism*. Berkeley: University of California Press.

Johnson, Barry. 1992. *Polarity Management: Identifying and Managing Unsolvable Problems*. Middleville, Mich.: Polarity Management Associates (PMA).

Jones, Daniel. 2004. *The Bastard on the Couch: Twenty-Seven Men Try Really Hard to Explain Their Feelings about Love, Loss, Fatherhood, and Freedom*. New York: Morrow.

Kipnis, Laura. 2003. *Against Love: A Polemic*. New York: Pantheon.

Kleinplatz, Peggy, ed. 2001. *New Directions in Sex Therapy: Innovations and Alternatives*. New York: Brunner-Routledge.

Love, Patricia, and Jo Robinson. 1995. *Hot Monogamy: Essential Steps to More Passionate, Intimate Lovemaking*. New York: Plume.

Levine, Stephen, ed. 2003. *Handbook of Clinical Sexuality for Mental Health Professionals*. New York: Brunner-Routledge.

Maltz, Wendy. 1992. *The Sexual Healing Journey: A Guide for Survivors of Sexual Abuse*. New York: HarperPerennial.

McDougall, Joyce. 1995. *The Many Faces of Eros: A Psychoanalytic Exploration of Human Sexuality*. London: Free Association.

Miller, Michael Vincent. 1995. *Intimate Terrorism: The Crisis of Love in an Age of Disillusion*. New York: Norton.

Mitchell, Stephen A. 2002. *Can Love Last? The Fate of Romance over Time*. New York: Norton.

Morin, Jack. 1995. *The Erotic Mind*. New York: HarperCollins.

O'Connor, Dagmar. 1986. *How to Make Love to the Same Person for the Rest of Your Life and Still Love It*. London: Virgin.

Ortega y Gasset, José. 1992. *Études sur l'amour*. Paris: Éditions Payot et Rivages.

Pasini, Willy. 1997. *La Force du désir*. Milan: Arnoldo Mondadori.

Paz, Octavio. 1995. *The Double Flame: Love and Eroticism*. San Diego, Calif.: Harvest.

Person, Ethel Spector. 1999. *Dreams of Love and Fateful Encounters: The Power of Romantic Passion*. New York: Penguin.

Person, Ethel Spector. 2002. *Feeling Strong: The Achievement of Authentic Power*. New York: Morrow.

Person, Ethel Spector. 1999. *Sexual Century*. New Haven, Conn.: Yale University Press.

Phillips, Adam. 1996. *Monogamy*. New York: Vintage.

Reibstein, Janet, and Martin Richards. 1993. *Sexual Arrangements: Marriage and the Temptation of Infidelity*. New York: Scribner.

Rubin, Lillian. 1990. *Intimate Strangers: Men and Women Together*. New York: HarperPerennial.

Saint-Exupéry, Antoine de. 1943. *The Little Prince*, trans. by Richard Howard. New York: Harcourt.

Salomé, Jacques. 2002. *Jamais seuls ensemble: Comment vivre à deux en restant différents*. Québec: Éditions de l'Homme.

Salomon, Paule. 2003. *Bienheureuse infidélité*. Paris: Éditions Albin Michel.

Salomon, Paule. 1994. *La Sainte Folie du couple*. Paris: Éditions Albin Michel.

Schnarch, David. 1991. *Constructing the Sexual Crucible: An Integration of Sexual and Marital Therapy*. New York: Norton.

Schnarch, David. 1997. *Passionate Marriage*. New York: Holt.

Semans, Anne, and Cathy Winks. 2004. *Sexy Mamas: Keeping Your Sex Life Alive While Raising Kids*. Maui: Inner Ocean.

Shernoff, Michael. 2006. *Without Condoms*. New York: Routledge.

Stein, Joseph. 2004. *Fiddler on the Roof: Based on the Sholom Aleichem Stories*. New York: Limelight Editions. (Reprint of original script, 1965. New York: Pocket Books.)

Steinberg, David, ed. 1991. *Erotic by Nature: A Celebration of Life, of Love, and of Our Wonderful Bodies*. Santa Cruz, Calif.: Red Adler/Down There.

Steinberg, David, ed. 1992. *Erotic Impulse: Honoring the Sensual Self*. New York: Tarcher.

Stoller, Robert J. 1985. *Observing the Erotic Imagination*. New Haven, Conn.: Yale University Press.

Stoller, Robert J. 1979. *Sexual Excitement : Dynamics of Erotic Life*. New York: Pantheon.

Tiefer, Leonore. 1995. *Sex Is Not a Natural Act and Other Essays*. Boulder, Col.: Westview.

Articles

Amatenstein, Sherry. 2005. "The Romance Is Disappearing from Our Marriage." *Redbook,* October, pp. 100–04.

Bass, Barry A. 2001. "The Sexual Performance Perfection Industry and the Medicalization of Male Sexuality." *Family Journal: Counseling and Therapy for Couples and Families,* 9, pp. 337–40.

Bass, Barry. 2002. "Behavior Therapy and the Medicalization of Male Sexuality." *Behavior Therapist,* 26, pp. 167–68.

Baumeister, Roy F. 2004. "Gender and Erotic Plasticity: Sociocultural Influences on the Sex Drive." *Sexual and Relationship Therapy,* 19, pp. 133–39.

Bender, Michele. 2005. "Twelve Resolutions for an Incredible Sex Life." *Redbook,* October, pp. 104–08.

Linda Berne and Barbara Huberman. "European Approaches to Adolescent Sexual Behavior and Responsibility: Executive Summary and Call to Action." Washington, D.C.: Advocates for Youth, 1999.

Bridges, Sara K., Suzanne H. Lease, and Carol R. Ellison. 2004. "Predicting Sexual Satisfaction in Women: Implications for Counselor Education and Training." *Journal of Counseling and Development,* 82, pp. 158–66.

Cherlin, Andrew J. 2004. "The Deinstitutionalization of American Marriage." *Journal of Marriage and Family,* 66, pp. 848–61.

Clements-Schreiber, Michele E., and John K. Rempel. 1995. "Women's Acceptance of Stereotypes about Male Sexuality: Correlations with

Strategies to Influence Reluctant Partners." *Canadian Journal of Human Sexuality,* 4, pp. 223–34.

Dunne, Gillian A. 2000. "Opting into Motherhood: Lesbians Blurring the Boundaries and Transforming the Meaning of Parenthood and Kinship." *Gender and Society,* 14, pp. 11–35.

Ellis, Bruce J., and Donald Symons. 1990. "Sex Differences in Sexual Fantasy: An Evolutionary Psychological Approach." *Journal of Sex Research,* 27, pp. 527–55.

Fisher, Helen E., Arthur Aron, Debra Mashek, et al. 2002. "Defining the Brain Systems of Lust, Romantic Attractions, and Attachment." *Archives of Sexual Behavior,* 31, pp. 413–19.

Flanagan, Caitlin. 2004. "How Serfdom Saved the Women's Movement: Dispatches from the Nanny Wars." *Atlantic Monthly,* March, pp. 109–28.

Flanagan, Caitlin. 2003. "The Wifely Duty." *Atlantic Monthly,* January-February, pp. 171–81.

Gafni, Mordechai. 2003. "On the Erotic and the Ethical." *Tikkun Magazine,* April–May.

Glade, Aaron C., Roy A. Bean, and Rohini Vira. 2005. "A Prime Time for Marital/Relational Intervention: A Review of the Transition to Parenthood Literature with Treatment Recommendations." *American Journal of Family Therapy,* 33, pp. 319–36.

Goldner, Virginia. 2004. "Review Essay: Attachment and Eros—Opposed or Synergistic?" *Psa Dialogues,* 14(3), pp. 381–96.

Heiman, Julia R., and John P. Hatch. 1980. "Affective and Psychological Dimensions of Male Sexual Response to Erotica and Fantasy." *Basic and Applied Social Psychology,* 1, pp. 315–27.

Hiller, Dana V., and William W. Philliber. 1986. "The Division of Labor in Contemporary Marriage: Expectations, Perceptions, and Performance." *Social Problems,* 33, pp. 191–201.

Hoggard, Liz. 2005. "Brooke Shields Talks about Strength, Truth and Love." *Redbook,* pp. 117–21.

Jamieson, Lynn. 2004. "Intimacy, Negotiated Nonmonogamy, and the Limits of the Couple." In *The State of Affairs: Explorations in Infidelity and Commitment,* eds. Jean Duncombe, Kaeren Harrison, Graham Allan, and Dennis Marsden. Mahwah, N.J.: Lawrence Erlbaum Associates, pp. 35–57.

Jarvis, Louise. 2005. "Love: What Makes It Last." *Redbook*, September, 205, pp. 160–65.

Julien, Danielle; Camil Bouchard, Martin Gagnon, and Andrée Pomerleau. 1992. "Insiders' View of Marital Sex: A Dyadic Analysis." *Journal of Sex Research*, 29, pp. 343–60.

Jung, Willi. 1997. "The Significance of Romantic Love for Marriage." *Family Process*, 36, pp. 171–82.

Kleinplatz, Peggy J. 1996. "The Erotic Encounter." *Journal of Humanistic Psychology*, 36, pp. 105–23.

Kleinplatz, Peggy J. 1992. "The Erotic Experience and the Intent to Arouse." *Canadian Journal of Human Sexuality*, 1, pp. 133–39.

Kleinplatz, Peggy J. 2001. "On the Outside Looking In: In Search of Women's Sexual Experience." *Women and Therapy*, 24, pp. 123–32.

Kleinplatz, Peggy J. 2003. "What's New in Sex Therapy? From Stagnation to Fragmentation." *Sexual and Relationship Therapy*, 18, pp. 95–106.

Kleinplatz, Peggy J., and Alia Offman. 2004. "Does PMDD Belong in the DSM? Challenging the Medicalization of Women's Bodies." *Canadian Journal of Human Sexuality*, 13, pp. 17–27.

Leiblum, Sandra Risa. 2002. "Reconsidering Gender Differences in Sexual Desire: An Update." *Sexual and Relationship Therapy*, 17, pp. 57–68.

Leiblum, Sandra Risa. 2003. "Sex Starved Marriages Sweeping the U.S." *Sexual and Relationship Therapy*, 18, pp. 427–28.

Leiblum, Sandra Risa. 1990. "Sexuality and the Midlife Woman." *Psychology of Women Quarterly*, 14, pp. 495–508.

Leiblum, Sandra Risa. 2001. "Women, Sex, and the Internet." *Sexual and Relationship Therapy*, 16, pp. 389–405.

Linn, Ruth. 1995. "Thirty Nothing: What Do Counselors Know about Mature Single Women Who Wish for a Child and a Family?" *International Journal for the Advancement of Counselling*, 18, pp. 69–84.

Liu, Chen. 2003. "Does Quality of Marital Sex Decline with Duration?" *Archives of Sexual Behavior*, 32, pp. 55–60.

Lobitz, W. Charles, and Gretchen K. Lobitz. 1996. "Resolving the Sexual Intimacy Paradox: A Developmental Model for the Treatment of Sexual Desire Disorders." *Journal of Sex and Marital Therapy*, 22, pp. 71–84.

Lykins, Amy D., and Marta Meana. 2004. "Book Reviews: The Science of

Romance: Secrets of the Sexual Brain." *Archives of Sexual Behavior,* 33, pp. 515–22.

Malamuth, Neil M. 1996. "Sexually Explicit Media, Gender Differences, and Evolutionary Theory." *Journal of Communication,* 46, pp. 8–31.

McCarthy, Barry. 2001. "Male Sexuality after Fifty." *Journal of Family Psychotherapy,* 12, pp. 29–37.

McCarthy, Barry. 2003. "Marital Sex as It Ought to Be." *Journal of Family Psychotherapy,* 14, pp. 1–12.

McCarthy, Barry. 1999. "Marital Style and Its Effects on Sexual Desire and Functioning." *Journal of Family Psychotherapy,* 10, pp. 1–12.

Merkin, Daphne. 2000. "The Last Taboo." *New York Times,* December 3.

Montgomery, Marilyn J., and Gwendolyn T. Sorell. 1997. "Differences in Love Attitudes across Family Life Stages." *Family Relations,* 46, pp. 55–61.

Nichols, Margaret. 1987. "What Feminists Can Learn from the Lesbian Sex Radicals." *Conditions: Fourteen,* ed. Conditions Collective. New York, pp. 152–63, 159.

Ogden, Gina. 2001. "The Taming of the Screw: Reflections on 'A New View of Women's Sexual Problems.'" *Women and Therapy,* 24, pp. 17–21.

Ogden, Gina. 1988. "Women and Sexual Ecstasy: How Can Therapists Help?" *Women and Therapy,* 7, pp. 43–56.

Pacey, Susan. 2004. "Couples and the First Baby: Responding to New Parents' Sexual and Relationship Problems." *Sexual and Relationship Therapy,* 19, pp. 223–46.

Parker, Lynn. 1999. "Bridging Gender Issues in Couples Work: Bringing 'Mars and Venus' Back to Earth." *Journal of Family Psychotherapy,* 10, pp. 1–15.

Person, Ethel Spector. 1986. "Male Sexuality and Power." *Psychoanalytic Inquiry,* 6. pp. 3–25.

Person, Ethel Spector. 2004. "Personal Power and the Cultural Unconscious: Implications for Psychoanalytic Theories of Sex and Gender." *Journal of the American Academy of Psychoanalysis and Dynamic Psychiatry,* 32, pp. 59–75.

Person, Ethel Spector. 1993. "Psychoanalytic Theory of Gender Identity." *Psyche,* 47, pp. 505–29.

Person, Ethel Spector. 1980. "Sexuality as the Mainstay of Identity: Psychoanalytic Perspectives." *Signs,* 5, pp. 605–30.

Philaretou, Andreas G., and Katherine R. Allen. 2001. "Reconstructing Masculinity and Sexuality." *Journal of Men's Studies,* 9, pp. 301–21.

Rampage, Cheryl. 1994. "Power, Gender, and Marital Intimacy." *Journal of Family Therapy,* 16, pp. 125–37.

Reibstein, Janet. 1997. "Rethinking Marital Love: Defining and Strengthening Key Factors in Successful Partnerships." *Sexual and Marital Therapy,* 12(3), pp. 237–47.

Scheinkman, Michele. 2005. "Beyond the Trauma of Betrayal: Reconsidering Affairs in Couples Therapy." *Family Process,* 44, pp. 227–44.

Snyder, Douglas K., Donald H. Baucom, and Kristina Coop Gordon. 2004. "An Integrative Intervention for Promoting Recovery from Extramarital Affairs." *Journal of Marital and Family Therapy,* 30, pp. 213–31.

Snyder, Douglas K., Donald H. Baucom, and Kristina Coop Gordon. 2004. "Treating Affair Couples." *Clinical Psychology: Science and Practice,* 11, pp. 155–59.

Sperry, Len, Insoo Kim Berg, and Jon Carlson. 1999. "Intimacy and Culture: A Solution-Focused Perspective: An Interview." In *Intimate Couple.* Philadelphia, Pa.: Brunner/Mazel, pp. 41–54.

Talmadge, Linda. 1986. "Relational Sexuality: An Understanding of Low Sexual Desire." *Journal of Sex and Marital Therapy,* 12, pp. 3–21.

Tepper, Mitchell S. 1999. "Letting Go of Restrictive Notions of Manhood: Male Sexuality, Disability, and Chronic Illness." *Sexuality and Disability,* 17, pp. 37–52.

Tiefer, Leonore. 1996. "Towards a Feminist Sex Therapy." *Women and Therapy,* 19, pp. 53–64.

Tiefer, Leonore. 2001. "Arriving at a New View of Women's Sexual Problems: Background, Theory, and Activism." *Women and Therapy,* 24, pp. 63–98.

Tiefer, Leonore. 2002. "The Emerging Global Discourses of Sexual Rights." *Journal of Sex and Marital Therapy,* 28, pp. 439–44.

Tiefer, Leonore. 2004. "Offensive against the Medicalization of Female Sexual Problems." *Familiendynamik,* 29, pp. 121–38.

Tiefer, Leonore. 2000. "Sexology and the Pharmaceutical Industry: The Threat of Co-Optation." *Journal of Sex Research,* 37, pp. 273–83.

Tiefer, Leonore, and Heather Hartley. 2003. "Taking a Biological Turn: The Push for a 'Female Viagra' and the Medicalization of Women's Sexual Problems." *Women's Studies Quarterly,* 31, 42–54.

Waite, Linda J., and Kara Joyner. 2001. "Emotional Satisfaction and Physical Pleasure in Sexual Unions: Time Horizon, Sexual Behavior, and Sexual Exclusivity." *Journal of Marriage and Family*, 63, pp. 247–64.

Weil, Susanna M. 2003. "The Extramarital Affair: A Language for Yearning and Loss." *Clinical Social Work Journal*, 31. (1), 51–61

Welty, Ellen. 2004. "Give Your Marriage a Big Pick-Me-Up." *Redbook*, August, p. 138.

Wilson, Pamela M. 1986. "Black Culture and Sexuality." *Journal of Social Work and Human Sexuality*, 4, pp. 29–46.

Weingarten, Kathy. 1991. "The Discourses of Intimacy: Adding a Social Constructivist and Feminist View." *Family Process*, 30, 285–305

Wynne, Lyman C., A. R. Wynne. "The Quest for Intimacy." *Journal of Marital and Family Therapy*, 12, pp. 383–94.

Zimmerman, Toni Schindler, Kristen E. Holm, Katherine C. Daniels, and Shelley A. Haddock. 2002. "Barriers and Bridges to Intimacy and Mutuality: A Critical Review of Sexual Advice Found in Self-Help Bestsellers." *Contemporary Family Therapy*, 24, pp. 289–311.

Index